Intermittent Fasting 16/8

The Beginners Guide for Rapid Weight Loss with Intermittent Fasting Science - Perfect for Women and for Men - Very Fast When Combined with Ketogenic Diet

© Copyright 2019 by _____ All rights reserved.

This content is provided with the sole purpose of providing relevant information on a specific topic for which every reasonable effort has been made to ensure that it is both accurate and reasonable. Nevertheless, by purchasing this content, you consent to the fact that the author, as well as the publisher, are in no way experts on the topics contained herein, regardless of any claims as such that may be made within. As such, any suggestions or recommendations that are made within are done so purely for entertainment value. It is recommended that you always consult a professional prior to undertaking any of the advice or techniques discussed within.

This is a legally binding declaration that is considered both valid and fair by both the Committee of Publishers Association and the American Bar Association and should be considered as legally binding within the United States.

The reproduction, transmission, and duplication of any of the content found herein, including any specific or extended information will be done as an illegal act regardless of the end form the information ultimately takes. This includes copied versions of the work, both physical, digital, and audio unless express consent of the Publisher is provided beforehand. Any additional rights reserved.

Furthermore, the information that can be found within the pages described forthwith shall be considered both accurate and truthful when it comes to the recounting of facts. As such, any use, correct or incorrect, of the provided information will render the Publisher free of responsibility as to the actions taken outside of their direct purview. Regardless, there are zero scenarios where the original author or the Publisher can be deemed liable in any fashion for any damages or hardships that may result from any of the information discussed herein.

Additionally, the information in the following pages is intended only for informational purposes and should thus be thought of as universal. As befitting its nature, it is presented without assurance regarding its prolonged validity or interim quality. Trademarks that are mentioned are done without written consent and can in no way be considered an endorsement from the trademark holder.

Tables Of Contents

Introduction 1

Chapter One: What is Intermittent Fasting 16/8 4

Chapter Two: Benefits of Intermittent Fasting 26

    Increased Weight Loss 27

    Increased Longevity 31

    Human Growth Hormone Production 37

    Benefits to the Brain 40

    Fasting and Cancer 44

Chapter Three: How to Eat with Intermittent Fasting 50

    Vegetables 61

    Fruits 64

    Dairy 67

    Proteins 69

    Whole Grains 72

    Starches 73

    Oils and Seasonings 74

Chapter Four: Non-Fasting Day Recipes 77

    Breakfast 77

    Lunch 88

Dinner 98

Snacks 110

Chapter Five: Supercharge your Weight Loss 116

Breakfast 126

Lunch 126

Dinner 127

Keto Snacks 129

Chapter Six: Extras 141

Hydration 141

Coffee 144

Tea 146

Decaf vs. Caffeine 153

Exercise 157

Tips specific to 16/8 Intermittent Fasting 159

Conclusion 163

Introduction

Congratulations on the purchase *Intermittent Fasting 16/8* and thank you for doing so.

The following chapters in this book will introduce you to the world of intermittent fasting! Take a closer look at the science behind intermittent fasting and how it can completely change your life. Intermittent Fasting is a great way to feel healthier, lose weight, and improve overall health and wellness. So why not get into it?

Get ready to explore some tasty meals that cater to weight loss and wellness on days when you aren't fasting as well as what kinds of meals can be consumed on your intermittent fasting days. This book will take you down the path of getting started with your intermittent fasting meal plan.

Learn how the Intermittent Fasting 16/8 process can be effective on its own, but also when used in conjunction with Low Carb diets like the Ketogenic diet. Intermittent Fasting is great for both men and women. Don't let some of those gender-based books or articles turn you away because intermittent fasting has benefits for everyone!

There are many books on the market that discuss intermittent fasting, so I am pleased you decided to give this one a chance! Every effort was made to ensure it is full of as much useful information as possible; please enjoy! The goal of this book is to help you decide if Intermittent Fasting is the best meal plan for you, as well as give you the details you need to get started with your new lifestyle! Explore and Enjoy!

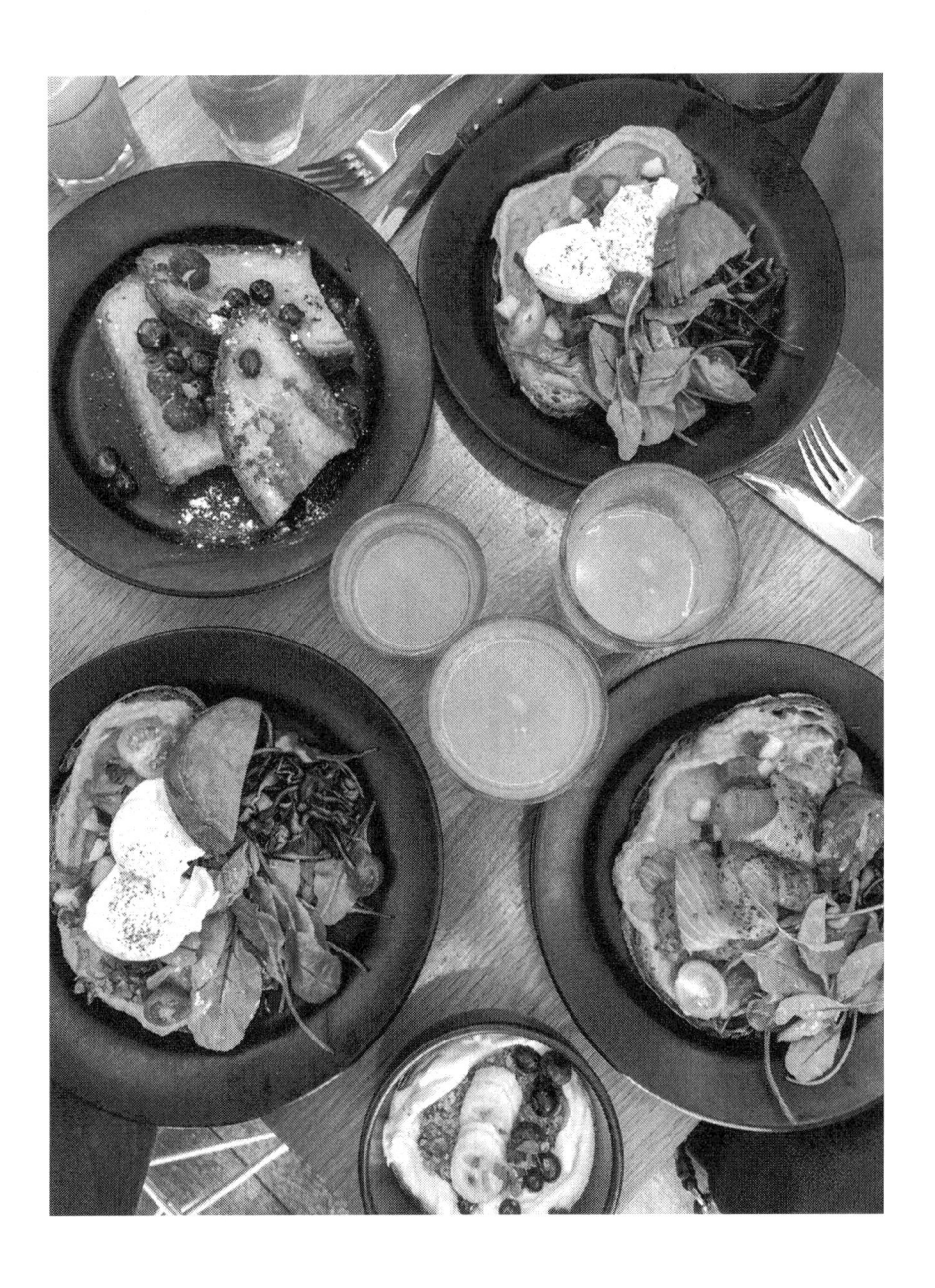

Chapter One: What is Intermittent Fasting 16/8

What makes the body healthy? In basic terms, being healthy is when the body is free of illness and injury. Both those ideas are pretty vague, however. Illness doesn't necessarily have to mean doctors, medications, and a stuffy nose. The injury doesn't have to be a scraped knee, a broken leg, or a fall on the ice. There are more subtle forms of illness and injury, and a lot of times they either go unnoticed in the body or are ignored because they are subtle.

If the joints have too much pressure on them, from sitting at a desk all day, or too much extra weight, that can be an injury that most people come to live with every day. So, in terms of health, having a constant injury, even if it is subtle and a result of your everyday job or lifestyle, it still means the body is not in optimal health.

Illness comes in a lot of forms as well. Some are easier to manage, and others might not be considered a problem. Sometimes, it isn't so much about a current illness as it is about keeping the body in a perpetual state that could later lead to more serious illness, such as chronically high blood sugar levels leading to Type 2 Diabetes. While high blood sugar levels may not impact everyday life, the body is essentially unhealthy as it has the potential to lead to illness.

With so many potential health risks that easily go unnoticed, how is anyone supposed to maintain their health and keep their body going? Well, there are a lot of diet and exercise plans available, and most do have their benefits. When thinking of potential lifestyle changes that could optimize the body's health, looking for a method that can be beneficial on many levels is sometimes the best way to go.

A major contributor to health, wellness, and weight is food. Everyone needs to eat. Food provides us with vitamins, minerals, protein, and the nutrients that keep our bodies healthy and functioning right down to a cellular level.

In most major societies, food is everywhere. There are large supermarkets filled with all kinds of food, Farmer's Markets with locally grown foods, big stores like Walmart and Target with grocery sections. There are restaurants, fast food, and food trucks. Even stores like bookstores and drugstores have snacks and candy readily available.

Sometimes it seems that eating is based less on hunger and based more on situations. When waiting in line at a drugstore, a chocolate bar can look very appealing! Long day at work and the idea of making a home cooked meal seems daunting; the fast food place around the corner is convenient and cheap! Going out with friends for a social visit, why not go out for coffee, and then have snacks on the side?

With constantly having food around us, and not all of it being very healthy, it is so easy to get sucked into unhealthy eating habits. Improper eating habits can cause several health-related issues.

Health issues from improper eating can include:

- Being overweight
- Being underweight
- Decreased immune system
- High blood pressure
- Candida Overgrowth
- Migraines

And several other health and body issues. The amount of food that is consumed, whether it is too much or not enough, is equally as important as the quality of the food being consumed. Unfortunately, poor quality food tends to induce a delicious flavor. Take fast food; for instance, greasy hamburgers are known to be unhealthy, especially ones from popular fast food joints. They are known to be covered in preservatives too, which make them harder to digest. Yet, they can be tasty! They are also convenient and cheap.

How is anyone supposed to eat healthily and keep their body healthy based on food and eating of unhealthy options are so easy to come by? The science behind a process known as Intermittent Fasting takes a look at just how to do that! So many diets require you to cut out all the delicious, and sometimes unhealthy, foods that you enjoy and that your body can even crave!

It can be so hard to stick to a diet when your body is telling you that you want to eat bread or that you don't want to stop putting sugar in your coffee. Additionally, most foods that are excluded from certain diets do, in fact, offer some nutritional benefits that the body needs. Even sugars and fats have an important role to play for a healthy, functioning body.

So then, how is it possible to lose weight, maintain bodily health, and also keep eating the foods you enjoy? Believe it or not, it is possible! One of the appeals to intermittent fasting is that it isn't a diet! It is a restricted eating schedule.
What exactly is fasting, and how can it produce rapid weight loss results?

What is fasting? Well, the dictionary says that fasting is when you willingly abstain from all food, drink, or both, or when you reduce your intake of food, drink, or both, for a designated period of time. There are different kinds of fasting, of course. Dry Fasting is the concept of complete abstinence from consuming all foods and drinks for a period of time. Intermittent Fasting is the process of alternating between periods of eating and fasting.

So then, what is the difference between fasting and starvation? Starvation is an involuntary process in which someone is denied food, or there is no food available. Fasting and intermittent fasting differ because they offer control. Control is one of the key components in making a fasting or intermittent fasting plan work.

There are many reasons for fasting, as well. Some people fast for religious traditions, body cleanses, and yes for weight loss and health. The Intermittent Fasting phenomenon is geared towards weight loss as well as boosting metabolic health, which helps protect the body from disease. There are some studies to indicate that Intermittent Fasting can contribute to increases in the average life span.

For thousands of years, different forms of fasting have been used throughout cultures across the world! This has all led to today's new varieties of fasting, including 16/8 Intermittent Fasting.

Gaining popularity across the country and the world, it is an easy form of fasting that has been said to be convenient and sustainable when trying to lose weight and improve health and wellness.

Right now, there are several variations on intermittent fasting. Some are more popular and have received media attention.

Some of the popular Fasting Plans include:

- **16/8 Intermittent Fasting**

  The basis is fasting for a 16 hour period and then consuming meals in a designated 8 hour period. During the 16 hours of fasting, no calorie and low carb beverages can be consumed, especially water.

- **5:2 Diet**

  During the week, select 2 days to eat only about five hundred to six hundred calories. The other five days in the week food can be consumed normally.

- **Eat-Stop-Eat**

For one or two days a week over a full 24 hour period, don't eat anything. Outside of those 24 hours, food can be consumed normally.

This book is primarily going to cover the 16/8 intermittent fasting plan and some additional information on how the Keto diet can be used alongside this fasting plan for increased weight loss benefits.

The basic idea behind the 16/8 intermittent fasting is that there are certain time periods for fasting, in which only unsweetened, low carbohydrate beverages can be consumed. These include water, coffee, and tea without any sweeteners or additives mixed in.

When considering how to optimize weight loss, but not necessarily wanting to stick to a strict diet, the 16/8 intermittent fasting plan is one to consider. Intermittent fasting relies on the body's ability to process fat stores during fasting cycles and then being conscious of the number of calories and carbohydrates being consumed during non-fasting cycles.

While it isn't required to give up any favorite foods for the 16/8 intermittent fasting plan, better results can be achieved when combining the intermittent fasting with a diet such as the Keto Diet or being more aware and conscious of the types of foods being put into the body. Luckily, since food is so accessible, that means healthy food is also accessible.

Farmer's Markets, natural food stores, even the big box grocery stores have healthy food and organic food sections. Sometimes these foods can be a little more costly. So here is another benefit of the 16/8 intermittent fasting plan. You eat less when restricting your meals to a specific time frame, as with intermittent fasting. It stands to reason that with eating less, you need to buy less food.

Buying less food means spending less money, or having more money to spend on healthier, better quality foods. With limiting the number of meals being eaten, that can free up personal time. Fewer meals lead to less time prepping meals.

Not only is this cyclical eating beneficial to weight loss and fat reduction, but it can impact the genes and hormones in the body as well as brain function, overall wellness, and longevity. Healthy cells and healthy hormone levels reduce the risk of illness on a short term basis as well as long term developments. Don't think of 16/8 Intermittent Fasting as a diet. It is more of a lifestyle. Lifestyle changes tend to be more effective than strict diets and firm exercise routines. Lifestyle changes allow for variation and flexibility and don't necessarily mean you have to give up everything you enjoy, just take a closer look at what and how you are incorporating them. In this particular instance, food.

It is easier to follow a healthy lifestyle when you don't have to force yourself to avoid certain foods or rearrange your schedule to include rigorous workout routines. With the 16/8 Intermittent fasting plan, many participants have reported feeling more energetic during fasting periods. With more energy, starting a new exercise routine could be a lot easier once you've gotten into the habit of intermittent fasting.

Limiting what you allow yourself to eat can also mean you have to miss out on certain activities, such as going out to eat with friends and family if the restaurant they are going to doesn't meet the dietary requirements you are trying to follow. Frustration with missing out and having to limit your food choices can lead to 'cheating' or completely giving up.

This is one of the reasons for utilizing a lifestyle plan like 16/8 intermittent fasting can be much more successful. Intermittent fasting is based on timing, not what can and can't be eaten.

That being said, in relation to food, consuming lower carb foods, or limiting your caloric intake during non-fasting times is the best way to ensure that your experience all the fine benefits of intermittent fasting, especially weight loss.

Now, in many societies, food is so easily and readily available. Because food and eating have become such an ingrained part of larger societies and cultures, the door has opened for food to be over consumed or even abused for emotional compensation.

Turning to an intermittent fasting lifestyle can help retrain the brain in eating habits. While eating can still be social, choosing when and how much to eat means that proper nutrition is attained and you leave behind a lifestyle of eating for the sake of eating.

Food is still available. Food will most likely always be available, but making a conscious choice of when to eat and how much you need to eat gives you the control to enjoy an intermittent fasting lifestyle. That being said, having a lack of control is one of the main reasons people tend to undereat, binge eat, or eat emotionally.

Taking control of food consumption and eating provides a sense of security and even empowerment. Unfortunately, seeking that control can sometimes lead to debilitating eating disorders. Here, intermittent fasting is a healthy alternative. It provides control, promotes the formation of healthier eating habits, and produces a lifestyle that encourages nutritional and health benefits.

While the idea of fasting and restricted eating might seem a little strange, think about how you might already incorporate intermittent fasting into your daily life. Do you have set meal times and limit the number of snacks you eat in between? When there is a period of time between meals that is intermittent fasting.

Do you have dinner and then not eat anything until breakfast the next morning? That is another fasting time. The term breakfast is a combination of the words 'break' and 'fast' because when you wake up after sleeping for 8 hours, you break your fast with a morning meal.

Sixteen hours a day are spent in this fasting cycle with the 16/8 intermittent fasting plan. Then for eight hours a day, meals and snacks can be eaten. There aren't any foods that are strictly off limits, but supercharging weight loss for more rapid results is best achieved if also following a low carb diet like the Keto diet.

Reasons to consider adopting a 16/8 intermittent fasting lifestyle include:

- Wanting to lose weight rapidly
- Need to lower blood sugar
- Build up insulin resistance
- Desire to improve overall health and wellness
- Control and empowerment over your body

So what happens when you fast? What happens to the body that makes fasting effective for weight loss?

When fasting, the body responds to the extended periods of time without food or caloric intake. One of the changes that the body experiences in fasting periods are changes in the cell functions, genes, and even hormones.

The cells react to fasting by entering an important repair process. During this process, waste material is removed from the cells. That waste material is unused fat stores that build up during non-fasting times.

Some of the changes that the body experiences on a hormone level are blood levels in the human growth hormone increases. This boosts the fat burning process and helps facilitate the muscle gaining process.

During fasting cycles, the genes themselves change in their expression. Genes and molecules that are known to be related to protecting the body against disease as well as longevity experience beneficial changes.

Another hormonal benefit the body experiences during intermittent fasting cycles is a significant drop in insulin blood levels. This drop increases the body's ability to burn fat.

Of course, the 16/8 intermittent fasting benefit that this book is mostly targeted towards is weight loss and cutting back on belly fat.

When operating on the intermittent fasting 16/8 cycle, it leaves less time for eating. This, in turn, generally means you will be eating fewer meals and thus fewer calories are being eaten in a given day. Fewer carbohydrates are consumed in a day if following the Keto Diet incongruence.

With the hormone changes in the body that are geared towards fat burning and break down, fat is turned into a main source of energy within the body. The metabolic rate is increased by short term or cyclical fasting because of the increased fat burning. The metabolic rate can increase by as much as 14% to assist with weight loss and calorie burning.

Between reducing the calories being consumed daily in congruence with a boost in metabolism, 16/8 intermittent fasting actually attacks weight loss from two angles.

Fasting has been known to decrease oxidative stress on the body. A decrease in oxidative stress reduces inflammation and also reduces the risk of chronic diseases.

There have been reviews on intermittent fasting data that suggest intermittent fasting can be responsible for up to an 8% rate of weight loss over the course of up to twenty-four weeks. This is a considerable rate of weight loss. The data also indicated that the people who had been monitored for this scientific data review exhibited up to 7% loss in waist circumference. This data would suggest that they lost a great deal of belly fat.

Belly fat can accrue in the abdomen and become harmful, causing or contributing to disease.

When dieting to burn fat, sometimes the diets can also start to reduce muscle mass and tone if not properly balanced with exercise. Intermittent fasting has been known to cause less reduction in muscle mass than other calorie restricted diets.

With all this scientific information and the data reviews of people that have tried intermittent fasting, it is easy to see how and why intermittent fasting can work so well towards weight loss, fat burning, and reducing waist circumference.

So we've covered some of the scientific evidence that backs up how intermittent fasting changes the body to achieve weight loss, but how does it work? On a scientific level, how does the fasting process allow the body to change and reap such wonderful benefits?

There is science to suggest that when the body fasts, even for a period of sixteen hours, the cells in the body begin to experience stress. This kind of stress isn't necessarily a bad kind of stress. Mild stress to the cells can cause them to adapt and enhance their resistance in an effort to protect the body. This resistance can increase the body's effectiveness in fighting and preventing disease.

Compare intermittent fasting to rigorous exercise. Rigorous exercise stresses the muscles and even the cardiovascular system. As long as the body is given ample time to heal and recover between exercise routines, then muscle tone and mass begin to increase, and the body becomes stronger.

Intermittent fasting can have similar results in the body. Mildly causing stress creates the environment within the body that is needed to produce the health benefits people are achieving with intermittent fasting! Then the body is allowed to 'rest' and 'heal' during nonfasting periods before the stress is induced again.

Taking a look at digestion, the digestive process breaks carbohydrates from food down into sugars. These sugars can be used by the cells as energy sources. They are essentially the gas, the powers, and the cells for cellular function. If your cells are provided with too much glucose and can't break it all down, that glucose gets stored as excess fat.

When the body is fasting, no carbohydrates are being provided for the cells to use as energy. Glucose stops being the main fuel source for cell function, and the cells then turn to fat stores for energy. Burning through fat stores is what ultimately contributes to weight loss.

Consuming fewer carbohydrates prevents excess fat stores from building up again. That is why intermittent fasting and the Keto Diet work so well together. Ketogenic diets are based around consuming fewer than 20 carbohydrates a day.

Intermittent fasting should not be painful or cause suffering. If you are underweight and do not have enough body fat stored, intermittent fasting can lead to undesired results and even painful outcomes. The intention is to promote health and wellness, including weight loss, not starve or malnourish the body.

Healthy weight loss is important when taking care of the body. It is possible to lose weight rapidly and remain healthy. Finding the balance and control between fasting and proper nutrition is why intermittent fasting allows you a safe and effective way to achieve a target weight.

It is important to remember that even with intermittent fasting, the overall goal is to reduce the number of calories being consumed a day by restricting when food can be eaten. If you are interested in following a 16/8 intermittent fasting plan, there is a danger to binge eating once the fasting period has ended. Overconsumption of calories has the potential to undo the benefits the body receives from the fasting cycle.

The body might take some time to adjust to an intermittent fasting cycle. The first few days might be harder, and your body might feel hungrier. Anytime you make lifestyle changes, especially ones that directly impact the body, you'll feel it.

There are some other potential risks with starting an intermittent fasting lifestyle. Sometimes, while the body is adjusting, you can experience dizziness, nausea, and periods of low blood sugar, or even the desire to eat more. Drinking plenty of water during fasting periods can help reduce these risks.

If you have a history of eating disorders, intermittent fasting may not be the best choice. The restricted eating time can encourage a binging habit during eating cycles or a purging habit during fasting cycles.

Additionally, there is some evidence to suggest that intermittent fasting may not be ideal for women as it has the potential to affect men and women differently. Some animal studies have shown that intermittent fasting can interfere with fertility in females. This has not been tested with humans, but there is always the potential for risk.

If you decide that this is the right lifestyle change for you, start slowly and gradually. If you experience any negative symptoms, it is recommended that you consult a doctor or health professional. The same goes for any concerns that might arise when you are starting your new intermittent fasting plan.

Before deciding to pursue an intermittent fasting diet, consider some instances in which intermittent fasting may not be the best choice.

Intermittent fasting may not be right if you are:

- Suffering from any chronic fatigue condition
- Suffering from HPA axis dysregulation
- A woman who is trying to get pregnant or maximize fertility
- Suffer from or have suffered from any eating disorders
- Are under a great deal of stress

In many aspects of life, finding the balance between two opposing ends is important. The same goes for dieting, food, and weight loss, fasting, and feeding.

So, we have seen the science to back up why intermittent fasting can and does provide great weight loss and health benefits. We have covered how it impacts the body and why the fasting cycle produces the benefits that people seek. This chapter has reviewed different kinds of fasting as well as how to optimize the benefits of intermittent fasting.

This chapter also discussed some of the risks that can be involved in an intermittent fasting plan isn't used correctly or without the proper information.

The following chapters of this book are going to go into greater detail of the benefits of intermittent fasting on the 16/8 plan. They will provide you with tips on how to get started and what kinds of foods should be prominent in your new lifestyle. There will be sections of this book that contain recipes for you to get started with, specifically Keto based recipes to ensure minimal carbohydrate intake.

While this is a beginner's guide to starting a 16/8 intermittent fasting lifestyle, by the end, you should have all the information you need to venture into your new intermittent fasting lifestyle!

While restricted eating and intermittent fasting do have some potential risks, they have also become quite popular, and there is plenty of scientific evidence to back up the benefits. There are hundreds of success stories and scientific data to support why the 16/8 intermittent fasting plan can and does promote weight loss, health, and wellness.

Are you now considering taking the 16/8 Intermittent Fasting cycle for a test drive? If not, keep reading! If you are, keep reading! Take this opportunity to really read about how to take control of your health, the benefits that stand to be gained from intermittent fasting, and how to start forming healthier eating habits.

Empower yourself with the knowledge that rapid weight loss and fantastic bodily health can be achieved without running yourself ragged with intense exercise. Learn how timing is all it really takes to start your weight loss journey.

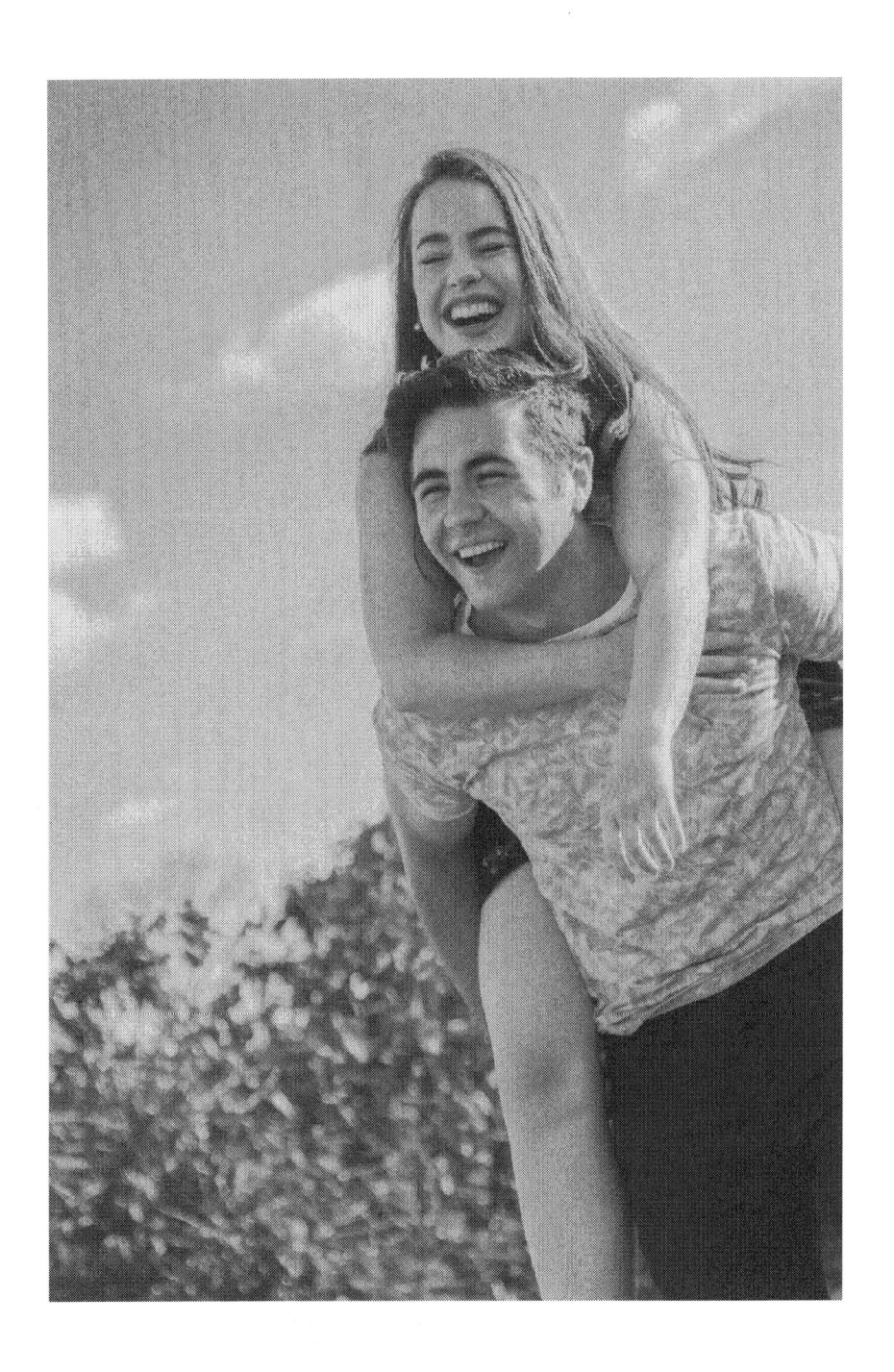

Chapter Two: Benefits of Intermittent Fasting

What is the point of intermittent fasting? Well, that's easy. The primary reason that people start to take an interest in intermittent fasting is for rapid weight loss. And why not? Many individuals, both male and female, do struggle with maintaining healthy weights.

Is that the only reason to try intermittent fasting? Absolutely not! Intermittent fasting can provide the body with several benefits. Some of these benefits are felt and seen in day to day life, like weight loss, losing belly fat, and reduction of inflammation. Yet, there are benefits that work on a more long term scale.

Studies have shown that following an intermittent fasting cycle reduce blood sugar levels, reducing the risk of blood sugar related complications. Additional studies have shown that intermittent fasting has the potential to reduce the risk of Alzheimer's disease.

So, intermittent fasting can help with both short term and long term health! The results can be rapidly noticeable, as well.

The following chapter is going to be a breakdown of the benefits from the 16/8 intermittent fasting plan with the scientific details as to why the body responds in those ways.

Increased Weight Loss

Okay, so you've tried diets for weight loss before. What makes Intermittent Fasting different from all the other diets that have come and gone? Well, first of all, Intermittent Fasting isn't a diet; it is a lifestyle! Get that notion of 'diet' of the brain. A lot of people hear or read the word 'diet,' and they immediately discredit the information.

Now that we have moved past the concept of 'diet' and are sticking to the idea of a lifestyle, what makes the 16/8 Intermittent Fasting plan ideal for weight loss?

Well, 16/8 refers to the fact that in 24-hour days, 16 hours of the day are spent fasting and 8 hours are allotted for meals and snacks. That may not seem like much, but between full-time work schedules, getting the kids to and from school, visiting friends and family, eight hours can fly right by!

Generally, a popular time cycle for the 16/8 intermittent fasting lifestyle is scheduling the fasting time to include the 8 or so hours you spend sleeping.

So, the non-fasting eight hours is most popularly scheduled during the workday. It can be difficult to eat more than one large meal during a work shift. Therefore, while following this popular schedule, most people will skip a morning meal, have a large afternoon meal with some snacks before and after and then forgo a large evening meal or have a smaller evening meal.

One large meal and some snacks throughout an 8 hour period will tend to consist of far fewer calories and carbohydrates than eating three big meals and additional snacks. That in itself is a start to the weight loss process and one of the reasons the 16/8 intermittent fasting plan can be so effective.

What happens when we consume food? Well, digestion is a rather complex process, but the part that is relevant to an intermittent fasting cycle is how carbohydrates from food are transformed into glucose. Glucose feeds the cells of our bodies, giving them the energy to carry out their designed function.

While cells do need glucose to power themselves, they aren't high-performance machines. A car can only drive so many miles on a gallon of gas. The rest of the gas in the tank just hangs around until it can be used. Cells can only burn through so much glucose at a time.

When eating bigger meals and snacks, the body has the potential to take in far more carbohydrates than the cells can process. Unlike a car gas tank, the cells don't just hold onto the glucose until it can be used. Excess glucose gets turned into fat stores in the body, contributing to weight gain and belly fat accumulation.

Without restricting eating times or allowing for fasting cycles, the body cells are likely to default to the fresh, new glucose being provided every time a meal or snack is consumed. Whatever glucose has become a fat store is just going to sit there unnoticed, accumulating more fat.

Looking back at intermittent fasting, when the body isn't taking in more carbohydrates to become glucose, the cells don't stop functioning. Cells continue to work and do their jobs, but they still need fuel. So they turn to other fuel sources. These sources are the accumulated fat stores.

So why is the 16/8 intermittent fasting cycle ideal? Well, the body can take up to 10 hours to start processing its fat stores.

Fasting for 16 hours gives the body ample time to start processing fat stores and burn through a portion of them.

Great, so we know how fasting contributes to weight loss and how restricting the eating time contributes to weight loss. Well, how do they work together? Why is the 16/8 intermittent fasting plan better than the other options out there?

The theory is, when the body fasts for 16 hours, it is able to burn through fat stores. Then when food is consumed for 8 hours in smaller portions and with fewer calories and carbohydrates, the fat stores don't build up at the same rate they are being burned. As you can see, this method if fasting ensures that the fasting cycle and non-fasting cycle both contribute to weight loss.

Looking at some of the other plans, if you fast for 2 days a week, during those 48 fasting hours, plenty of fat can be burned, but nothing restricts you from replenishing those fat stores the other 5 days during the week.

As you can see, a continuous cycle of intermittent fasting, like the 16/8 cycle can ensure maximum weight loss because it approaches the issue from two angles.

Now consider the Keto Diet. Ketogenic diets are based on the concept of the body only consuming about 20 Carbohydrates a day. This is stricter than just following an intermittent fasting cycle; however, it can really supercharge weight loss!

Carbohydrates provide the cells with Glucose. The keto diet can kick weight loss up a notch because, during the 8 hours of non-fasting, fewer carbohydrates mean less fat going into storage. It also means that by the time you enter your fasting cycle, the cells might already be looking for more fuel, so it could take less than 10 hours for them to start burning through fat stores.

The 16/8 Intermittent Fasting plan provides a multi-faceted approach to weight loss and fat burning, encouraging greater success. The weight loss process can be expedited by following a low carb diet alongside your fasting cycle.

Increased Longevity

The idea of living longer is popular in many societies. Pharmaceutical companies develop medications to reduce aging side effects. Cosmetic companies created lotions and creams to reduce and reverse wrinkles. Hair salons work with a lot of clients who color their hair regularly to hide grey and white as aging changes hair color. To more extreme levels, plastic surgeons provide services such as Botox and body modifications that provide a younger, firmer appearance.

People want to live longer.

However, after all, said and done, plastic surgery, medications, and cosmetics don't really stop the body from aging. Bodies do age, and no one has come up with a cure for an age yet.

That doesn't mean increasing personal longevity and lifespan are fantasies that are out of reach. In fact, intermittent fasting has been known to aid in increased longevity! How strange is that? Actually, it isn't as odd as it sounds.

Intermittent Fasting and restricted eating plans do have something in common. Whether you are intentionally counting calories or just carefully following your 16/8 intermittent fasting plan, calories do tend to get restricted when eating and fasting this way.

Good news! Caloric restriction has reportedly been the most efficient way to combat aging!

How does Calorie Restriction combat aging? Well, the aging process is about as complex as the human body itself. That is to say; it is very complex. Aging isn't fully understood in the scientific community, just like the human body. There is always more to learn, but what we do know now is that restricting calories impact five mechanisms that contribute to human aging. Caloric restriction supports these five mechanisms in a way that promotes much healthier and longer aging cycles.

The five mechanisms that caloric restricting impacts are:

- Cell Proliferation
- Mitochondrial Physiology
- Inflammation
- Antioxidants
- Autophagy

I know, those sound pretty heavy in terms of scientific terminology. Fortunately, all five of these mechanisms are interrelated with each other and in human aging.

Cell proliferation is also referred to as Growth Balance. When cells are in an anabolic state, they are powered up for building organs and tissues. Cells remain in an anabolic state when there is an abundant supply of calories, like when we eat regular meals and snacks.

With regular fasting and caloric restriction, cells are allowed to enter their catabolic state. Cells in a catabolic state are breaking down, recycling, and repurposing tissues.

Allowing the body proper cycles to break down and repurpose old tissues and then cycle into building up new tissues perpetuates a healthy cycle of regenerating tissues, thus provided longer life to organs and body tissues.

Mitochondria are parts of cells. They are organelles that are needed to create ATP or cellular energy. This ATP allows the cells to work and powers cells in both physical and cognitive labor.

As the body ages, it starts to impair mitochondrial network quality. When the network quality diminishes, the breakdown of damaged and dysfunctional mitochondria is decreased as is the body's ability to build new mitochondria.

Intermittent fasting and caloric restriction help both the destruction and creation of damaged and new mitochondria, respectively.

Animal studies have shown that since cells are exposed to less glucose during fasting, the ATP production does drop off for a while. This triggers a process in the cell to replenish ATP and allow cells and mitochondria to better produce ATP in the future. Kind of like a computer reboot but of the ATP production in a cell.

As the body ages, joints and other body parts begin to experience damage from use and wear and tear over the years. To protect the body, the immune system begins to create inflammation. In itself, inflammation is not bad as it is a natural protective response the body has to injuries.

Unfortunately, as the body ages, damage and injury accumulate and become more prevalent. In an attempt to protect itself, the immune system keeps producing inflammation, sometimes contributing to chronic inflammatory diseases.

Fasting and calorie restriction has an inhibiting effect on one of the nuclear factors that exert anti-inflammatory effect. Basically, reducing this nuclear factor's (Nf-kB) activity through calorie restriction forces the signals in the immune system that create inflammation under-regulated, producing less inflammation. Less inflammation means the aging body is less prone to chronic inflammatory issues.

Intermittent fasting and calorie restriction help antioxidant defenses. During the aging process, reactive oxygen species increase and antioxidant defenses decrease. As this imbalance grows, damage accumulates (creating inflammation) and mitochondria begin to malfunction faster (mitochondrial physiology).

Trying to balance the reactive oxygen species with antioxidant defenses helps with mitochondria function and preventing chronic inflammation. That's where intermittent fasting and calorie restriction comes into play again! Calorie restriction promotes antioxidant defenses by activating nuclear factor (Nrf2), which regulates the cell's ability to resist oxidants.

In regards to autophagy, which translated at its root words quite literally means 'self-eating. As autophagy progresses, old cell structures and cell junk are removed. This junk can accumulate over time and hinder cells from performing at their highest level. This is where fasting and growth hormone become beneficial.

During a fasting cycle, the human growth hormone is amplified and kind of on overdrive. When this hormone kicks on, it signals the body to produce replacement parts for the pieces that are being scrapped during autophagy. This includes mitochondria.

Autophagy is basically a recycling process for the cellular structures in the body. Since it relies heavily on growth hormone to actually recycle and repurpose the old, junky parts, then having growth hormone in an amplified state is beneficial to the process.

Here you can really see how these different mechanisms are interrelated. Thus, using intermittent fasting to restrict calories has a widespread benefit over the aging process and contributes to longevity.

Human Growth Hormone Production

Human growth hormone was touched on as being an important part of cell growth and regeneration through autophagy. The human growth hormone is vastly important to the body in other ways than just keeping the cells replenished and functioning smoothly.

The human growth hormone is produced in the pituitary gland in the brain. Levels of human growth hormone are higher in the body when children are growing. These levels peak during puberty, when the body goes through its most drastic hormonal changes. After puberty, the human growth hormone begins to dwindle in the body. This is normal in adults, but that doesn't mean the hormone isn't still beneficial.

The human growth hormone is suppressed during non-fasting periods because its function is to increase the blood glucose level. When calories and carbohydrates are being consumed, the human growth hormone goes on standby.

Fasting periods stimulate the secretion of the human growth hormone. This hormone is beneficial as it has a positive influence on the muscles, encouraging them to recover quickly. This specific benefit is important to anyone who is an athlete or exercises regularly.

Additionally, adults who are human growth hormone deficient tend to have higher levels of body fat and lower levels of lean body mass as well as less bone mass.

While all hormones are released periodically in the body naturally as a mechanism to prevent the body from building up a resistance, it is possible to have hormone deficiencies. That is why intermittent fasting can be beneficial in raising the growth hormone levels.

In as little as 5 days of fasting, the human growth hormone can have an increase of 300%. That is a lot in a short amount of time, so even in just 16 hours of fasting, human growth hormone production will go up.

As previously discussed, the human growth hormone helps in anti-aging, or healthy aging. It also helps the muscles recover for people who are athletes or regularly active. In one 6-month study of the human growth hormone in people, the group receiving hormone injections and the control group didn't exhibit differences in weight. However, the differences in lean mass vs. fat mass were quite noticeable.

Those receiving the human growth hormone injections increased their lean mass (muscle mass) by about 8.8 percent more than the control group. Their fat mass had an average 14.2% decrease and a loss of 5.3 lbs. of fat mass! The skin even exhibited thickening.

So, there it is, the human growth hormone can and does contribute to a reduction in fat mass and an increase in lean mass. This is great for anti-aging, but also anyone looking to decrease their body fat levels and increase their muscle mass. Of course, working out and exercising while intermittently fasting will also enhance muscle mass, especially with additional production of the human growth hormone.

Fasting is the best way to naturally stimulate the production of the human growth hormone. This hormone is crucial to child development, puberty, and continued functionality in the body into adulthood.

It doesn't take extensive fasting periods for the human growth hormone to start being produced. Therefore, sticking to the 16/8 intermittent fasting cycle will include the human growth hormone benefits.

Benefits to the Brain

Did you know that fasting can also be beneficial to brain health and longevity? It is incredible how many areas of the body fasting seems to impact in a positive way!

The brain is a highly complex structure in the body with endless functions and importance. It makes sense that we should take care of our brains then, right? Brain cells tend to grow slower than cells in the rest of the body. BDNF is a protein that plays a pivotal in the stimulation of growing new brain cells as well as the function of neurons.

BDNF is the equivalent to a brain growth hormone. Very important, very essential. Stimulating the BDNF protein is a highly valuable benefit for the brain.

Do you know what stimulates the protein BDNF? You guessed it, fasting! Fasting can supercharge the brain by stimulating the BDNF protein.

There is additional scientific research done on animals to suggest that intermittent fasting provides mice with better learning capacity and better memory. There is more evidence to suggest that intermittent fasting can reduce inflammation in the brain, which reduces risks to neurological conditions.

More studies have been done on animals in regards to intermittent fasting cycles that show a reduced risk of Alzheimer's disease, stroke, and Parkinson's disease.

Evolutionarily speaking, the human brain evolved to basically be a hybrid vehicle. Rather than running off of electricity and gas, the brain functions best when there is a metabolic transition between running on ketones and running on glucose. Brain cognition tends to be at its highest when switching metabolic functions.

That being said, intermittent fasting naturally enhances brain growth factors, growth of neurons, and neuroplasticity.

Neuroplasticity is essential to providing the brain with resistance to injury and disease, including degenerative and neurological diseases.

So here is an interesting take. True caloric restriction diets tend to encourage people to eat less than 1000 calories a day. There is a lot of feedback to indicate people who eat less than 1000 calories a day are hungry and uncomfortably craving food a lot.

Now consider the Keto Diet. Ketogenic restricts carbohydrate intake but not caloric intake. This is just another example of how the ketogenic diet can so greatly compliment an intermittent fasting lifestyle. Your body will get the calories it needs to be energized and full, but those fat store producing carbohydrates are limited.

Intermittent fasting does have calorie restricting attributes; however, it isn't essential to gain benefits. Now, allowing the body to be intermittently hungry, as in intermittently fasting, allows the brain and body to do what it naturally wants to do! While the body is burning fat during a fasting cycle, the ketones will keep the brain going and improve overall cognition.

Additionally, ketones will improve the growth and connections between neurons and build up resistance to neurological and degenerative brain diseases. Intermittent fasting allows the brain to complete its own natural cycles of switching between metabolic processes.

Back in the days of hunter-gatherers, it was not uncommon for meals to be separated by 10 to 12 hours or even a few days. This was an early time in human evolution. Doesn't it make sense that the brain and body would evolve to accommodate proper bodily function and benefit during periods of time when food wasn't available?

Humans haven't evolved much on an anatomical or physiological level since then. However, societies have grown and changed, providing us with ever easier access to food and other commodities.

Our bodies and brains haven't quite caught up to our societies yet, in a way. Human bodies and brains still behave the same way, on a physiological level, as they did millions of years ago. Evolution is pretty neat. Due to evolution, our human bodies adapted to certain circumstances and environmental factors, like the potential space between meals.

Our bodies have everything they need to function properly and healthily. It is up to us to allow our bodies the time and nutrients to achieve the health standards that we are designed to reach!

There are some neurosurgeons who greatly advocate for the intermittent fasting meal plan. Their general consensus is to hit at least two 16 hour stretches fasting time every week. Again we see why the 16/8 intermittent fasting method is so beneficial. By default, it has those recommended 16 hour fasting periods!

Fasting and Cancer

For over a hundred years, the effects of fasting on cancer cells and calorie restriction have been researched. These studies have primarily been done on mice and animals. However, there are current trial studies being offered with humans to determine if the results are the same.

That being said, the data discovered in mice and animals would be highly impactful if the results are the same in people. A lot of the science behind why fasting works in animals should be the same in people, but the scientific data doesn't yet back it up officially.

Fasting is essentially denying yourself food. One of the reasons the body builds up a resistance to disease and illness during fasting times is because when the body isn't getting food, it adapts. Energy is diverted into different protective systems within the body to minimize the damage should the denial of food be prolonged. There is plenty of thought that these protective processes can help decrease the risk of cancer.

Fasting and calorie restriction without pushing the body into a malnourished state has been said to be one of the most potent physiological interventions to help prevent cancer and protect the body against cancer in mammals, which includes humans.

In a study done on rodents in regards to intermittent fasting and mammary tumors, the rodents experienced a 40 to 80 percent reduction in tumor incidences. That is a drastic difference!

Another theory states that cancer cells are not protected by the same protective signals that are stimulated when the body is fasting. The rest of the body is on lockdown, but the cancer cells are still 'exposed' giving the immune system and white blood cells a chance to attack and fight the cancer cells more effectively as well as improving results of cancer treatments. This protective state can also help in protecting mammalian cells, and human cells, from the destructive toxins in the chemotherapy.

It is said that fasting can help regenerate a stronger immune system. If the immune system has already been depleted by harsher treatments, intermittent fasting can assist in rebuilding that system to continue to combat the cancerous cells.

Eight different cancers were studied in mice in relation to intermittent fasting. The study showed that in five out of the eight cancers, intermittent fasting slowed the growth of the cancers. The study also demonstrated that intermittent fasting alongside chemotherapy treatments was more effective on all eight cancers that were studied.

For women, a recent study indicated that women who fasted for at least 13 hours a day, or overnight, reduced their chances of reoccurring breast cancer after treatment by 36 percent. This same study showed that these women were 21percent less likely to experience mortality due to breast cancer.

There it is, not only does intermittent fasting have the potential to decrease cancer risk, but it can also slow the spread of cancer and assist cancer treatments in fighting cancer. Additionally, it has the ability to protect the body from harmful side effects of cancer treatments like chemotherapy or radiation.

While the field of science is always changing, new studies with new results are always coming to light. It is important to discuss any concerns or questions with your health care provider or a professional in a specialized field if you would like to try to maximize your health benefits.

A lot of this science is new and still being studied more extensively in humans. There are trials running, and more current information is always coming to light.

That being said, the 16/8 intermittent fasting lifestyle has the potential to promote rapid weight loss, increase longevity, stimulate human growth hormone secretion, protect the brain and encourage optimal functionality, and decrease the risk of cancer and cancer growth.

Before switching to 16/8 intermittent fasting to treat, manage, or benefit any health condition, please consult your physician and allow them to guide you through the proper steps.

The human body is such an amazing machine! Knowing how it works means that we can keep finding more effective ways to maximize our health and functionality. Looking into evolution as well as smaller aspects like hormone secretion and protein stimulation gives us a better understanding of how to use the resources at our fingertips to keep ourselves ticking.

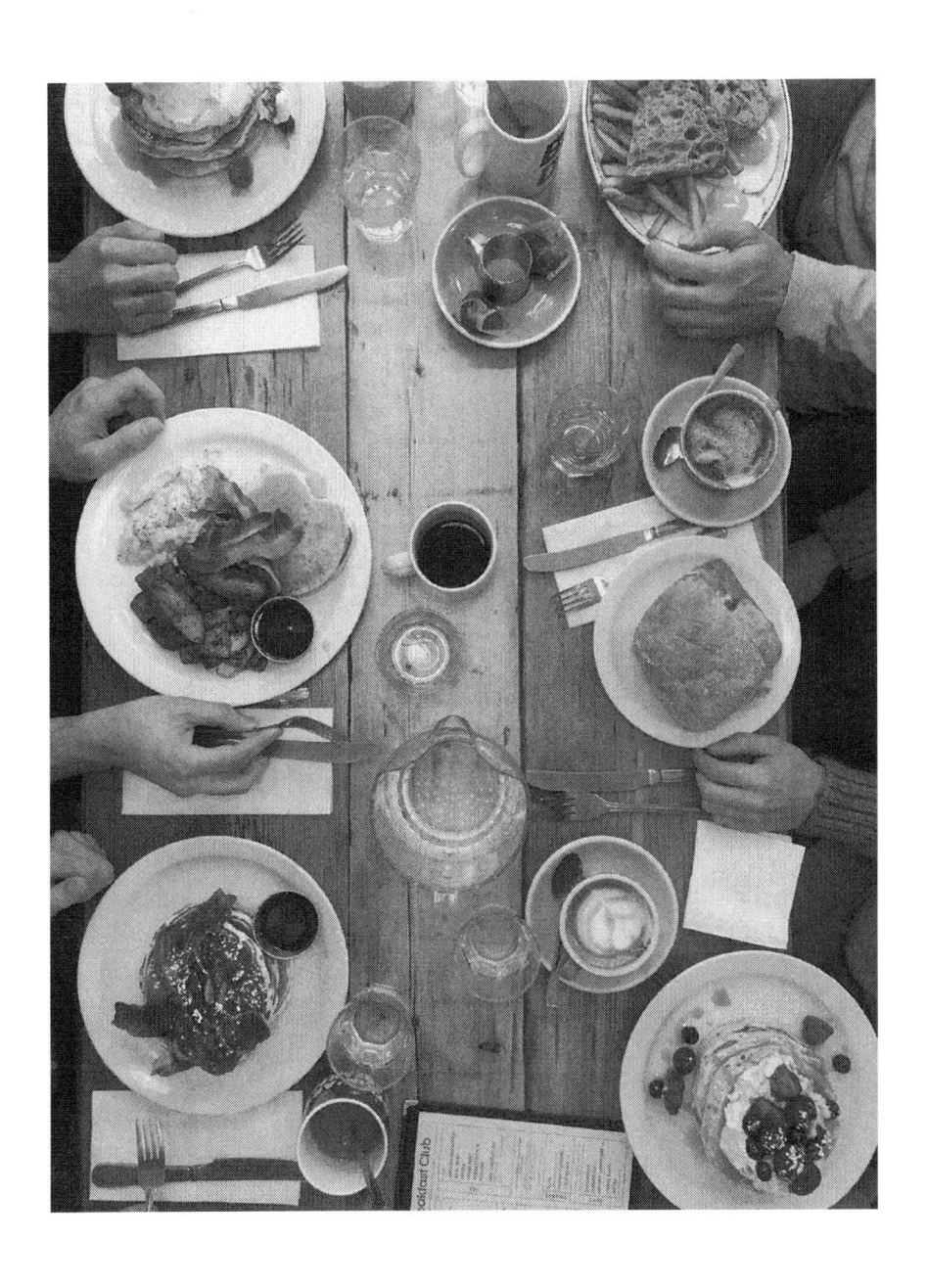

Chapter Three: How to Eat with Intermittent Fasting

Now that we know the basics of how to utilize an intermittent fasting method as well as many of the great benefits of intermittent fasting, it is time to talk about how to get the 16/8 intermittent fasting method working for you!

Let's backtrack for a moment. The 16/8 intermittent fasting method is when you spend 16 hours a day fasting and 8 hours a day is reserved for meals and snacks.

During a fasting cycle, you can drink water, unsweetened tea, and black coffee or other zero calorie and low carb beverages. Water is recommended to prevent dizziness, nausea, and other potential side effects while your body is adjusting to a fasting cycle. Drinking unsweetened, low-calorie beverages can also help curb your appetite, so you don't have as many cravings or a desire to binge after fasting.

While you are in an 8-hour non-fasting cycle, there are no foods that are strictly off limits. However, to supercharge weight loss and maximize the benefits of intermittent fasting, utilizing a diet like the Keto Diet, or other low carb diets can definitely help.

Okay, we've reviewed the basics, so what is the first step in starting to adopt and intermittent fasting lifestyle.

Well, the first step is to decide how you want to divvy up your time.

Most people who follow that 16/8 fasting method do try to schedule the 16 hours along with their sleep schedule. That way, they can sleep through a good portion of their fasting cycle.

Depending on when you go to sleep, that could be a factor for deciding when you'd like to schedule your fasting period.

As for the window for eating, there are some considerations. For example, does the company you work for offer free food regularly? If that is the case, it might be a good idea to make sure some of your eating time is during your work shift. Or are you someone with an active social life who likes to go out and enjoy dinner and drinks with friends? You don't want to miss out on that!

Everyone has a different lifestyle, but with the 16/8 intermittent fasting method, you have the power and control to decide when you want to eat, and what times are important for you to be able to eat.

A lot of people following this fasting lifestyle prefer to eat from 12:00 pm to 8:00 pm. This means skipping breakfast, but being able to enjoy lunch and maybe a small dinner, and then fasting overnight.

Another popular schedule is eating from 9:00 am to 5:00 pm as it sits in line with the average work schedule. This allows for breakfast and lunch with a light, small dinner. Then you still fast overnight.

It might be worth trying out a couple of different time schemes to see what really works best for your lifestyle.

Once you decide on the right timing, it might be a good idea to ease into intermittent fasting, especially if you've never tasted before. Easing in can mean you start with just following the cycle a couple of days a week and build up to following the intermittent cycle full time.

Another style for easing into intermittent fasting is to start by fasting for 12 hours, and once your body gets used to that, jump up to 14 hours. After your body acclimates to the 14-hour fasting, move up to the 16 hours of fasting, which is where you want to be.

Whatever works for your body and your schedule, and you'll know what makes sense for you. Easing in is an attempt to give your body time to adjust so you are less likely to experience dizziness or nausea. This will also continue to encourage healthy eating habits and avoid developing a binging problem if you feel like you are starving every time your non-fasting cycle comes around.

Regardless of what time frame you do go with, it is recommended that you space out meals and small snacks over the eight hours. This has two functions, to curb a potential binging habit by keeping your body satisfactorily full during those 8 hours. It also makes sure that you eat regularly enough, so you aren't feeling hungry by at the beginning of your fasting cycle. That could make 16 hours feel like a very, very long time.

It is worth noting that the body will take time to adjust. Don't give up! Let your body acclimate and give the intermittent fasting time to work. Barring surgery, there isn't really an instant weight loss fix. Thankfully there are noninvasive, less expensive options that also contribute to a well-rounded, healthy body.

When you are ready to start the intermittent fasting cycle, take into consideration some of the recommended food choices during your non-fasting cycle. Again, these are recommendations to help maximize your weight loss and body fat reduction!

Fruits: Berries, apples, oranges, bananas, peaches, grapes, etc.

Vegetables: Leafy greens, kale, broccoli, cauliflower, tomatoes, peppers, cucumbers, onions, mushrooms, root vegetables, etc.

Healthy Fats: Coconut, olive oil, avocados

Sources of Protein: Poultry, fish, eggs, lean red meat, eggs, nuts, and seeds, etc.

Dairy: Milk, yogurt, cheese, kefir, etc.

Whole Grains: Rice, barley, quinoa, buckwheat, ancient grains, etc.

Remember, if you are sticking to the Keto diet as well, avoid all grains, starchy vegetables like legumes, root vegetables, and corn, and stick to small portions of fruits like a few berries here and there. Also avoid alcohol, sugars, and sweeteners (unless they are low carb sweeteners). These carbohydrate-rich foods and beverages do not align with Ketogenic Diet requirements.

Below is a basic outline of an early eating window, midday eating window, and late eating window time frames for meals and snacks as well as some meal and snack suggestions. In the recipes section, there will be more detailed meal ideas to get you started!

Early Eating Window
8:00 am: Veggie omelet with Cheese

12:00 pm: Apple and Carrot slices with Peanut (or another nut) Butter (Substitute apples and carrots with celery sticks for Keto diet)

4:00 pm: Stir-fried veggies and chicken over a bed of Jasmine Rice (substitute the Jasmine rice for cauliflower rice on the Keto diet)

Evening: Decaf tea or decaf black coffee
Midday Eating Window
Morning: Black coffee or unsweetened tea

11:00 am: Yogurt and fruit smoothie (plain yogurt with berries for a Keto diet)

2:00 pm: Apple slices with cheese and quinoa crackers (cheese slices and sliced broccoli and bell peppers for Keto diet)

4:00 pm: Chia pudding with fruit topping (fruit topping optional for Keto Diet)

6:00 pm: Sweet chili turkey meatballs with whole wheat pasta (use zucchini pasta and low carb tomato sauce for Keto Diet)

Late Eating Window
Morning: black coffee or unsweetened tea

1:00 pm: Small leafy green salad with tomato, avocado, cucumber, and onion (dressing optional)

4:00 pm: Fresh broccoli, cucumber, bell pepper, and cauliflower slices with ranch dressing (Low Carb ranch for Keto Diet)

9:00 pm: Grilled fish filet with roasted root veggies and quinoa (substitute the root veggies with broccoli and bell peppers and the quinoa with cauliflower rice for Keto diet)

Making sure each snack and meal has sources of protein, calories, and carbohydrates, even in small amounts, helps keep the body going through the non-fasting period. Relying on clean, whole foods for nutrients is the best way to maximize your weight loss experience with intermittent fasting.

That's not to say you can't indulge in or enjoy some greasy food or treats now and then. Balance and moderation are the keys to success in any type of lifestyle change.

Tracking calories isn't necessary during your eating window. However, if your main goal is to lose weight, considering the calories and carbohydrates that are going into your body can help you reach your weight loss goals faster.

Going back to evolution, human bodies evolved in a hunter and gatherer lifestyle. Not only were large meals spread out over several hours based on food availability, but snacks and 'grazing' were a common practice.

Picking berries and eating them throughout the day, or foraging for vegetables and consuming them regularly helped keep human bodies strong and healthy between larger meals.

This ties directly back into the 16/8 intermittent fasting method where the absence of larger meals is supplemented by smaller but healthy snacks. Grazing is the idea that small amounts of food are consumed over long periods of time. Grazing can encourage bad eating habits.

Think of a pet dog. Most dogs that have self-refilling bowls are overweight. They see food is available, so they keep eating and eating. Humans trying to 'graze' can run into similar problems. A way to prevent unwanted over grazing habits to form is to fill your pantry or lunch bag with small, healthy snacks.
Carrot sticks, apple slices, grapes, cheese slices, celery, and peanut butter, mixed nuts, sunflower seeds, these are all examples of healthy snacks that can be casually nibbled on throughout the day, or in between larger meals without piling on the calories.

A lot of times, our bodies are full before they feel full. This can be caused by eating too quickly. The faster someone eats, the more food they can stuff into their stomach before the signal that indicates the body is full reaches the brain.
Here again, we see how eating small snacks at intervals throughout the day, or even grazing on healthy snacks can assist the body in intermittent fasting. Allowing the digestive system to receive the calories and nutrients and give it time to

process what is available without overloading it can help train the brain not to experience strong cravings.

During a non-fasting cycle, if there is a steady amount of calories, carbohydrates, and nutrients being provided, then those nagging hunger pains that make fasting and losing weight so difficult don't bother you.

So, during a non-fasting cycle, remember to stick to whole, clean foods as much as possible. Healthy nutrients, healthy fats, and healthy snacks. Plan to have one large meal or two smaller meals, and then supplement with nutrient-rich, healthy snacks at various intervals.

These steps will help train the body not to feel starved in between snack and meals by providing the proper nourishment to carry over to the next snack or meal. They will encourage the development of healthy eating habits. Most importantly, they will promote healthy weight loss and reduction of body fat.

On the subject of nutrients, there are many cultures that believe proper nutrients isn't extracted from food unless it is chewed between 30 and 50 times before being swallowed. The average adult human has 32 teeth in their mouth. These teeth are shaped differently for different uses. However, the mouth is where digestion starts!

Food should be chewed thoroughly so that saliva can help break it down and extract the right nutrients. Swallowing large chunks of food means the digestive system isn't able to break down the chunks properly and receive what nutrients are contained within the food.

If you are a fast eater, yet you are committed to intermittent fasting and losing weight, consider slowing down your eating. Consciously count the number of chews for each bite of food. Not only will this ensure you get the full nutrients every bite has to offer, but it will allow your body to feel full naturally. It will discourage binging and could even help your body adjust to the intermittent fasting cycle better.

Pavlov's Bell is a well-known scientific study in which Pavlov wanted to study conditioning responses. He would ring a bell and then feed his dogs. At the sight of food, dogs would begin to salivate. After a while of ringing the bell before feeding them, the dogs began to salivate at the sound of the bell rather than the sight of food.

Humans can also recondition themselves in similar ways. This is why intermittent fasting can be a little difficult to adjust to at first. Fortunately, the more you stick to it, the more your body and brain are reconditioned to know that you aren't being starved during a fasting period.

Let's talk more about food. What kinds of food should be in your pantry? Previously we listed some examples of the kinds of whole foods that are ideal during an intermittent fasting plan. Now we are going to go over some healthy options in each category as well as some not so healthy options.

Vegetables

There are a lot of available vegetables out there. Thankfully, they are usually a healthy option for meal sides and snacks. Vegetables can be used in many different ways for healthy eating.

Leafy greens, for example, have endless uses. Kale, spinach, arugula, bok choy, and collard greens are a few examples that make excellent additions to soups, stir-fries, salads, even smoothies! They are also an excellent source of Vitamin K and calcium. Having some leafy greens on hand is always a good idea. They are quite versatile and healthy!

Some favorite vegetables include:

- Broccoli
- Cauliflower
- Carrots
- Cucumbers
- Bell Peppers
- Onions
- Mushrooms
- Squash
- Beets

This is a generic list of vegetables that are useful as sides and/or snacks, so having a few readily available can make a meal and snack prep much easier!

In regards to the Keto diet, root vegetables are too full of carbohydrates to include in ketogenic meals. That includes carrots, parsnips, beets, radishes, turnips, and other starchy root veggies.

Of course, the list of vegetables is virtually endless, but there are some others that offer great health benefits and can be quite tasty!

A few of the more unique vegetables include:

- Brussel Sprouts
- Fiddle Heads
- Turnips
- Parsnips
- Radishes
- Artichokes
- Bean Sprouts
- Okra
- Asparagus
- Eggplant

Some of these vegetables, like fiddleheads and artichokes, do require special preparation, but that doesn't mean they are any less delicious or healthy!

The versatility of vegetables extends beyond what can be easily seen. Take cauliflower, for example. Cauliflower can be turned into a faux-mashed potato kind of side dish for anyone avoiding starches or on the keto diet. Cauliflower can also be made into a rice substitute for keto diet followers or anyone cutting back on grains.

For people who are gluten-free, following the keto diet, or just trying to cut back on carbs and grains, Spaghetti Squash is a great alternative. Cabbage and Zucchini can also be shredded into the past like a substitute.

Fruits

The fruit is a delicious snack! Full of natural sugars they can provide that fix for any sweet tooth craving. Fruit can be eaten alone as a snack, combined with other snack foods, and used as a topping to enhance meals.

Unfortunately, fruits can be high in carbohydrate; it's those natural sugars. If you are limiting carb intake or following the keto diet, it is best to stick to small portions of berries or avoid fruits altogether.

Its recommended that you have a variety of fruit available for health benefits, but also because they can be a very convenient snack on their own. No additional prep and don't usually require utensils to eat! Grab an apple and eat it on the go.

Favorite fruits to have on hand:

- Apples

- Bananas
- Peaches
- Berries (blueberries, strawberries, raspberries, blackberries, etc.)
- Pears
- Tomatoes
- Oranges
- Grapes

Any of the above fruits can be a snack on their own. Fruit salads are excellent, healthy snacks. Add some berries or apple slices to yogurt or top off your morning oatmeal with them.

Tomatoes are technically a fruit; however, they are more commonly seen paired with vegetables, in sauces, or in salads. However, a fresh, sliced tomato sprinkled with a little salt does make a fantastic snack!

Like vegetables, there are tons of less common fruits that can be enjoyed as well. Sometimes eating the same foods over and over can get boring. That can be a contributing factor as to why heavily restricted diets can lead to frustration and failure. How can you stick to a diet when you don't enjoy the eating?

Everyone should enjoy eating!

So as with vegetables, there are also some less common fruits that can bring variety, excitement, flavor, and enjoyment into your non-fasting cycles.

Some unique fruits are:

- Kiwi
- Mango
- Melon (Cantaloupe, Watermelon, Honeydew)
- Star Fruit
- Pomegranate
- Papaya
- Plum
- Kumquats

At a basic grocery store, it is pretty easy to find some of the more unique fruits out there. Fruits can be frozen to keep them longer.

Frozen berries and vanilla yogurt blended together make a wonderful breakfast smoothie! Frozen fruits can even be blended to make a dairy-free, healthier ice cream that isn't so full of sweeteners and processed flavors.

Dairy

Dairy can be a very healthy aspect of regular meals. There are a lot of people who struggle with the digestion of dairy. If you are one of those people, stick to what your body tells you in regards to dairy products.

Dairy can be consumed on the keto diet. It is low in carbohydrates but rich in protein. With the keto diet, a plain yogurt with a low carb sweetener added is the best option.

Yogurt makes a delicious breakfast with some berries or a little cinnamon. Small portions of yogurt can also be consumed as a snack. Melted cheese can top off almost any meal wonderfully, and cheese slices with fruit are a great snack! Dairy is also quite versatile in its uses.

Common dairy sources include:

- Milk
- Cheese
- Yogurt
- Butter

Butter is a source of fat, so best consumed in smaller quantities when looking out for calorie intake. Yogurt is a strong source of probiotics which encourages intestinal health and clear skin.

Incorporating Raw Dairy into your diet can also promote health and wellness. Raw milk, cheese, and butter made from raw milk. Raw milk is not available in every state. If you do have access to raw milk, it is encouraged that you look into the quality assurance of the farm and company that produces it to ensure proper safety precautions are being taken.

Dairy doesn't just have to come from cows either! Some people who have a sensitivity to cow dairy have found that they can digest goat milk and cheese as well as sheep's milk and cheese. Goat and Sheep dairy is another healthy dairy source.
There are a couple of lesser-known dairy options that have great health benefits as well. Kefir and Ghee are two dairy options that are gaining popularity.

Kefir is similar to yogurt with a different consistency, more like a smoothie. It can be drunk straight, like a beverage. Kefir is rich in protein and probiotics. It has been known to help with chronic skin conditions when consumed regularly. Anytime you are changing your eating style or habits, having additional, natural sources of probiotics can be a good thing.

Probiotics help with digestion and intestinal health. When switching to an intermittent fasting method and/or changing the types of food you eat, sometimes the body has trouble adjusting. Probiotics can ease the transition by keeping the digestive tract healthy and functioning at top performance levels.

Ghee is another unique dairy option. Ghee is generally made from cow's milk. It is a highly-clarified form of butter. It can be used as cooking oil or as an ingredient in dishes. Often times, people who have trouble digesting dairy can still handle Ghee.

Proteins

Protein comes in many forms and sources. Traditionally, meat and fish are common forms of protein. When looking to optimize weight loss, sticking to leaner meats is a good option. Trimming the fat off of meat before preparing is also a good idea, and avoiding consumption of skin from the meat will cut down on calories and sodium intake.

Meat is also encouraged on the keto diet. If following the keto diet, make sure to use low carb seasonings.

Common meat sources include:

- Red Meat
- Pork and Ham
- Chicken
- Salmon
- White Fish

These meats have many different applications from soups, to grilling, pan searing, and can be enhanced with glazes, marinades, and herb rubs.

Some leaner meat options that can offer variety and a good source of protein and vitamins are Bison, Venison, and Ostrich meat. These meats may not be as easily acquirable, but they do make a delicious meal!

Shellfish, such as crab, lobster, mussels, clams, and scallops, are also rich in protein and can be a fantastic source of protein.

While thinking about seafood and fish, it is best to avoid fish like swordfish and tuna, or at least eat them in very small amounts with limited frequency. Swordfish and tuna have high concentrations of mercury, and this can become a problem over time, especially for women in their reproductive years.

For anyone who doesn't eat meat, there are lots of meat alternatives for protein. Many of these sources also have healthy fats in them and provide other health benefits. They can also be eaten as snacks in most cases.

Alternative protein sources include:

- Eggs
- Nuts
- Seeds
- Legumes

When following the ketogenic diet, legumes are too starchy and carbohydrate-rich to qualify. However, eggs, nuts, and seeds are acceptable.

Protein, of course, is a huge requirement for any successful meal plan. Other than eggs, nuts, and seeds, most protein sources do require a certain amount of preparation and planning. This is why they tend to make a better option for larger meals.

Whole Grains

Whole grains offer many health benefits; however, they are high in carbohydrates and may contain gluten. If you are following the ketogenic diet, whole grains are meant to be avoided. If you are gluten-free for any reason, make sure to double check on which whole grains have gluten and which do not.

Healthy whole grain options include:

- Rice
- Buckwheat
- Quinoa
- Ancient Grains
- Barley

Whole grains can be used in soups, as a side dish, or as part of the main dish like stir fries. Quinoa can be used in salads too! Whole grains usually offer additional preparation and cooking, so unless they are being added to a salad, they are a good addition to large meals.

Grains like bread, pasta, and other processed kinds of wheat tend to be high in carbohydrates and not ideal for losing weight.

However, there are some vegetable, bean, and quinoa-based kinds of pasta that are great alternatives!

Starches

The term 'starches' in this context is in regards to whole foods that aren't necessarily unhealthy, but shouldn't be eaten in large quantities regularly, especially when weight loss is the main goal.

These starches do not align with the ketogenic diet as they are full of carbohydrates.

Starches include:

- Potatoes
- Yams
- Turnips
- Beets
- Carrots
- Parsnips
- Corn
- Legumes

Most root vegetables are starchy foods. Beans and lentils are also high in carbohydrates. While these foods can make tummy side dishes, salads, and snacks and can even be good sources of protein, it is recommended that their consumption be moderated. Eaten in small portions or less frequently.

Oils and Seasonings

Of course, we want our food to taste good! That means your pantry should have some healthy herb, spice, and seasoning options available.

Some of the healthiest seasonings that are also ketogenic friendly include garlic and ginger. These are popular flavors, but the health benefits from both are incomparable to many other seasonings out there! Fresh garlic and fresh ginger are definitely thee way to go.

Olive oil and coconut oil are both wonderful drizzles to add a little flavor to salads and side dishes. They can also be used to grease pans for cooking as a healthy alternative to the cooking spray. Olive oil is not a high heat oil and should only be used at low heat temperatures or not heated at all.

The lists provided above are a great starting point for you to begin changing your eating habits and getting into your 16/8 intermittent fasting lifestyle.

Hopefully, you now have enough information to start planning your ideal 16/8 intermittent fasting schedule. You should know the basic idea of how your non-fasting meals and snacks should be laid out. You should also have a good guide to start filling your pantry with healthy, whole foods that you can enjoy in various ways!

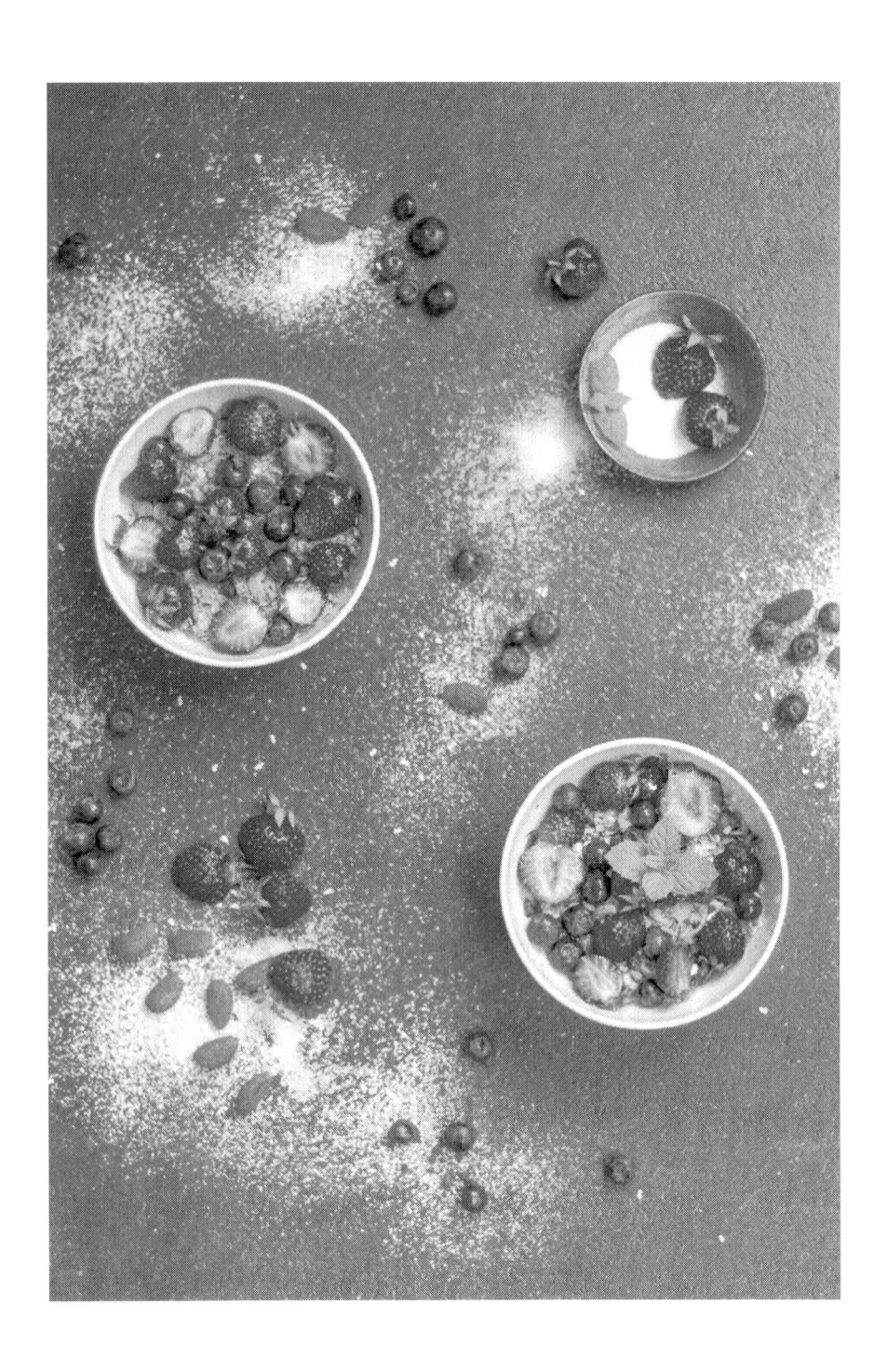

Chapter Four: Non-Fasting Day Recipes

In this chapter, recipes will be provided for breakfast, lunch, dinner, and snacks. That way, whatever eating window you decide to set for yourself, you will have a starting point. Any meals that are ketogenic friendly will be indicated as such.

Feel free to mix and match, and the start to make your own recipes! Half the fun is learning how to make healthier foods for yourself and make them tasty to your liking.

This is just a starting point for you to get going with your 16/8 intermittent fasting method and weight loss!

Breakfast

Breakfast Chocolate Shake (Keto)

Prep Time: Five Mins

Yields: One serving

Ingredients:

½ C coconut milk or heavy cream

½ C ice

One to Two tbsp. cocoa powder

½ medium avocado

Pinch of salt, Himalayan pink

Two to Four tbsp. erythritol or low carb sweetener of your choice

½ Tsp. vanilla extract

Optional Add-ins:

Ground chia seeds

Mint Extract

Hemp Hearts

Directions:

- Put all the ingredients into a blender, including any add-ins you want. Blend until creamy and smooth. Add in ice or additional milk to thin the consistency to desired thickness.
- Enjoy immediately!

Chocolate, Chocolate Chip Muffins (Keto)

Prep Time: Ten mins

Cook Time: Eleven mins

Yields: Eighteen little muffins

Ingredients:

One C almond butter, creamy

1/3 C confectioners erythritol (or preferred low carb sweetener)

Two tbsp. peanut butter powder

Two eggs, large

Two tbsp. cocoa powder, unsweetened

Two tbsp. filtered water

One tbsp. salted butter, melted (or coconut oil)

One tsp. baking soda

1 ½ tsp. vanilla extract

¼ C dark chocolate chips for baking, sugar-free

Directions:

- Start by preheating your oven to 350 degrees F. Set up a baking sheet with a mini muffin tin, silicone if you have it.

- Combine all the ingredients, except the chocolate chips, in a large mixing bowl and mix together by hand or with an electric mixer. Make sure to blend all the ingredients thoroughly. The mix should be thick and doughy.

- Now add the chocolate chips and fold them into the muffin mix.

- Fill eighteen mini muffin or twelve regular sized muffin slots about 2/3rd of the way full of the muffin mix.

- Set in the tray with the muffin pan on top in the oven and back at 350 degrees F for eleven mins. When the timer goes off, take the baking sheet and muffins from the oven.

- To check if they are cooked through, use a thin knife or toothpick, and poke down to the center of a muffin. If the knife or toothpick comes out clean, then they are cooked!

- Allow your chocolatey muffins to cool before enjoying them.

Spinach and Mushroom Omelet with Goat Cheese (Keto)

Prep Time: Five mins

Cook Time: Fifteen mins

Yields: One serving

Ingredients:

Two tbsp. olive oil

Three eggs

One C spinach

Two tbsp. goat cheese, crumble

Three Oz. preferred mushrooms, sliced

½ avocado, ripe and diced

Black pepper and salt

Fresh parsley, chopped

Directions:

- Heat olive oil in a medium-sized skillet on the stove over medium heat. Cook the mushrooms until they are tender and brown, this takes about five or six mins. Transfer the browned mushrooms from the stove to a bowl.

- Reheat the pan and coat with a little more olive oil. Whisk the eggs together and season with a bit of pepper and salt. Carefully pour the whisked eggs into the pan.

- Allow the eggs to cook until the edges start to set and the bottom browns. This will take approximately six to seven mins.

- Gently, using a rubber spatula, pull up the edges of the eggs to release them from the pan. Transfer them to a plate and lay flat.

- On half of the circular omelet set a layer of mushrooms, then spinach. Top with goat cheese and then the avocado slices. Fold the bare half of the omelet over the layered half and garnish with the fresh parsley. Enjoy warm!

Overnight Oatmeal

Prep Time: Five Mins

Cook Time: Eight Hours

Yields: One serving

    Ingredients:

    <u>The oats</u>:
    ½ C quick oats or rolled oats
    ½ C yogurt (optional)
    ½ C milk (One C if not using yogurt)
    1/8 teaspoon salt
    Sweetener of choice (stevia, truvia, honey, etc.)

    <u>Optional additives</u>:
    ½ C chopped fruit or berries
    One tablespoon chia seeds
    One to Two tablespoon peanut butter (or preferred nut butter)

Directions:

- In a mason jar or another container with a lid, combine all the ingredients together. Put the lid on securely, and the container until all the ingredients are well blended.

- Place the shaken jar into the refrigerator and let sit overnight.

- The next morning, take the jar out and stir everything together. Then enjoy!

Chocolate Banana Shake

Prep Time: Five mins

Cook Time: Three mins

Yields: Three servings

Ingredients:

Four bananas, frozen and cut into chunks
1 ½ C almond milk, vanilla
Two spoonful's creamy peanut butter, heaping

Two tbsp. unsweetened cocoa powder

Directions:

- Toss all the ingredients into a blender. Run the blender until all the ingredients are combined and smooth until creamy. If it is too thick, add a little more almond milk and blend to desired consistency.

Breakfast Pumpkin Spice Milkshake

Prep Time: Ten mins

Cook Time: Ten mins

Yields: One serving

Ingredients:

¾ cup vanilla almond milk (or any milk)
¼ cup pumpkin puree
½ cup old fashioned oats
¾ teaspoons pumpkin pie spice
½ frozen banana
One tablespoon maple syrup (or sweetener of choice)

Powdered cinnamon

Directions:

- Combine the pumpkin puree, maple syrup, pie spice, and milk in a bowl. Whisk them all together until well combined. Stir the oats into the mix and then cover the bowl and refrigerate the mixture overnight.

- The following morning, use a fork to crush the frozen banana into the pumpkin mix. Then transfer the mixture to a blender. Blend together until smooth and creamy. If you prefer a thinner consistency, add a little more milk until you get the thickness you want.

- Pour the smoothie into a glass and sprinkle a pinch of cinnamon over the top, then drink.

Egg and Ham Scramble (Keto)

Prep Time: Fifteen min

Cook Time: Twenty Min

Yields: Ten servings

Ingredients:

Sixteen Eggs

Two C ham cubes, fully cooked

Two C shredded cheese

2/3 C sour cream

½ C milk

1 ½ C potatoes, peeled and diced

½ C green pepper, chopped

½ red pepper, chopped

½ onion, chopped

Two tsp. canola oil

½ tsp. salt

¼ tsp. pepper

Directions:

- In a small saucepan cover the potatoes with water and bring to a boil on high heat. Once boiling, bring the heat to low and cover. Allow simmering ten to fifteen mins until tender. Drain the potatoes.

- In a skillet, warm some of the olive oil and sauté the onion and half of the peppers. Stir in the potatoes and half of the ham. Continue to sauté for about two to three min.

- In a blender, add the sour cream, milk, salt, eggs, and pepper. Blend together until well combined and smooth.

- Pour half of the blended eggs over the veggies in the pan. Stir periodically and cook over medium heat until the eggs are done. Sprinkle with half of the cheese and then remove to a serving bowl.

- Repeat the above process with the second half of the ingredients.

- Egg scramble can be kept in a sealed container in the refrigerator for up to five days.

Lunch

Kale and Citrus Salad

Prep Time: Five min
Cook Time: Twenty-five min

Yields: Six servings

Ingredients:

Salad
One bunch of Kale
One tbsp. olive oil
Large onion, chopped
½ C quinoa
One garlic clove smashed
½ C heaping, whole dates
½ C roasted almonds, salted or unsalted

Dressing
Juice of one clementine or mandarin orange
Juice of half a lime
¼ C olive oil
Sea salt and fresh ground black pepper
Two tbsp. real maple syrup

Directions:

- On the stove over medium heat, put the olive oil and chopped onion pieces into a sauté pan. Cook until the onion is nice and brown and caramelize. This should take about twenty mins. Take the onion off of the stove and set aside.

- Add the garlic and quinoa to a saucepan on the stove. Remember to rinse the quinoa with water before cooking. On the stove, set the heat to medium and toast the garlic and grain for once min. Then pour in a cup of water and bring to a boil.

- Cover the saucepan and set the heat to low, allowing to simmer for about fifteen mins. When the fifteen minutes are up, turn the heat off on the stove and let sit for five mins covered with the lid.

- Take the lid off the pot and use a fork to fluff up the grains.

- To prepare the kale, first, wash with cold water and let dry on a flat surface or use a paper towel to dry. Slice of the stems at the bottom. Cut the rest of the leaves into ribbon-like slices.

- Cut the pits out of the dates and cut the fruits into quarters. Chop the almonds up roughly. Now toss together the kale, quinoa, and onions.

- Mix up the dressing by combining the fruit juices, maple syrup, and olive oil. Whisk together until combined and then add a little pepper and salt. Mix half the dressing in with the salad greens and grains.

- Toss the salad with the dates and chopped almonds and add the remaining dressing if desired.

- This salad can be kept in the refrigerator for up to five days. It keeps well.

BLT Spring Rolls

Prep Time: Fifteen mins

Cook Time: Five mins

Yields: Four servings

Ingredients:

Roll Recipe

One tomato, seeded and sliced

Six bacon pieces, cooked crispy

Rice paper

Avocado slices

Fresh lettuce leaves, chopped

Fresh basil and mint, chopped

Dipping Sauce

¼ C filtered water, cold

One tbsp. mayonnaise

One tsp. sesame oil

One tsp. lime juice, freshly squeezed

¼ C soy sauce or tamari

One tsp. sriracha hot sauce

Directions:

- To make the spring rolls, fill a bowl with hot water and dip the rice paper into the water carefully, one wrapper at a time. Let them get damp for a few seconds and then take them out. Be careful not to oversoak them.
- Place the dampened wrappers on a plate or a flat working surface. The paper will become more pliable as it absorbs the water while sitting on the plate.

- To add the fillings, layer the bacon, lettuce, tomatoes, and avocado on 1/3rd of the rice paper. Roll the wrapper over the fillings, tucking the edges in and rolling carefully to make sure that the fillings are snug inside.

- To make the dipping sauce, combine all the sauce ingredients together in a small jar or blender. Tighten the lid on the jar and shake well to combine all the ingredients, or use the blender to mix them all together.

- Serve your spring rolls immediately. Serve the dipping sauce on the side, or drizzle the rolls with a little of the sauce before serving.

Burger with Guacamole

Prep Time: Ten mins

Cook Time: Twenty five mins

Yields: Four servings

Ingredients:

One lb. ground beef

Four burger buns

Four slices of pepper jack cheese

Two ripe Hass avocados

One jalapeno pepper, minced

Juice of one lime

¼ cup cherry tomatoes, diced

½ tsp. oregano, dried

Pinch of mustard seed, ground

Salt and black pepper

Directions:

- Put the ground beef in a bowl and season with salt, pepper, oregano, and ground mustard seed. Mix the seasonings into the beef well. Then portion the beef out into four hamburger patties.

- Light the grill charcoal or set the gas to high. Grill the burgers until they are pink, about six mins on each side at medium heat.

- Place one slice of cheese on each patty and let melt on the grill for about one min.

- While the burgers are cooking on the grill, mash the avocados in a bowl, then add in the tomatoes, lime juice, jalapeños. Mix together and season with a little pepper and salt.

- Set each burger on a patty and then top with a scoop of guacamole. Serve warm with roasted root vegetables on the side.

Guacamole Side Salad (Keto)

Prep Time: Ten mins

Cook Time: Five mins

Yields: Four servings

Ingredients:

Four C mixed salad greens
Six strips bacon, cooked and crumbled
Two ripe Hass avocados, peeled and cut into cubes
½ red onion, sliced into rings
Two tomatoes, seeded and diced
1/3 C olive oil

Two tbsp. apple cider vinegar

¼ tsp. hot pepper sauce

One teaspoon salt

¼ teaspoon ground pepper

Directions:

- In one bowl, mix the tomatoes, onions, and bacon. Stir together.

- In a separate bowl, combine the oil, vinegar, hot pepper sauce, salt, and pepper and whisk together until blended. Pour the sauce over the tomatoes, onions, and bacon.

- Now add the avocado cubes and mix together until the sauce coats the cubes. Next, toss the salad greens into the bowl with the other ingredients. Toss together to evenly coat everything.

Fruit and Yogurt Parfait

Prep Time: Five minutes

Cook Time: Five minutes

Yields: Four servings

Ingredients:

Three C vanilla yogurt
One C fresh or frozen strawberries (defrosted if frozen)
One C fresh blueberries (substitute raspberries or blackberries, or do a medley)
One C granola

Directions:

- Set out four glass jars. Layer 1//3 C of the yogurt in the bottom of each jar. Mix the berries together and add a layer over the yogurt. Then top with a layer of granola.

- Add a second layer of yogurt, berries, and granola, and then the jars are full. Serve immediately.

- If jars have lids, they can be refrigerated and stored for a few days (granola will lose its crunch if stored).

Dinner

<u>Meatballs and Pasta with Sauce (Keto)</u>

Prep Time: Twenty mins

Cook Time: Fifty mins

Yields: Four servings

Ingredients:

<u>Meatballs:</u>

One pound beef, ground

½ cup mozzarella cheese, shredded

¼ cup parmesan cheese, grated

One minced garlic clove

One egg, large and beaten

Two tablespoons fresh parsley, chopped

½ teaspoon black pepper, freshly ground

One teaspoon salt

Two tablespoons olive oil

<u>Sauce:</u>

28 ounces tomatoes, canned and crushed

One chopped onion

One teaspoon oregano, dried

Two minced garlic gloves

Salt and pepper

Spaghetti:

One medium spaghetti squash

Olive oil

Salt and pepper

Directions:

- Preheat the oven to 350 degrees F. Cut the spaghetti squash in half and spoon out the seeds, leaving as much of the flesh intact as possible. Brush the halves with olive oil and season with salt and pepper. Set the squash halves to face down on a baking sheet.

- Bake the squash for thirty to forty minutes.

- While the squash is baking, assemble the meatballs. Combine together the beef, cheeses, egg, garlic, parsley, and the salt and pepper. Mix the ingredients together well and then form sixteen meatballs by hand.

- Set a burner to medium heat and place a skillet over the burner. Heat the olive oil and then put the meatballs into the skillet. Turn them occasionally until the meatballs have become golden on all sides. It should take about ten mins.

- Remove the meatballs from the heat when they are golden and set on a plate that is lined with a paper towel.

- Use the same skillet to make the sauce. Soften the onion for five mins. Add in the garlic and sauté until deliciously fragrant, about one min. Mix the tomatoes, salt, pepper, and oregano into the pot.

- Once stirred, throw the meatballs back in the skillet with the sauce. Cover the pot and let the sauce and meatballs simmer for fifteen mins for the sauce to thicken.

- When the spaghetti squash is done in the oven, poke it with a fork to make sure it is tender. Allow cooling until it can be handled. Then use a fork to scrape out the flesh of the squash, and it will shred into squash noodles.

- Divide the squash noodles onto plates and top with scoops of sauce and meatballs. Sprinkle with a little parmesan cheese and then serve!

Grilled Salmon, Veggies, and Rice

Prep Time: Five mins

Cook Time: Ten mins

Yields: Four servings

Ingredients:

Salmon
1 ½ pound salmon, sliced into 4 smaller fillets
Olive oil

Seasoning
¼ cup of salt
¼ cup onion powder
¼ cup basil
¼ cup garlic powder
¼ cup dried parsley

Veggies

Two zucchinis halved and then quartered the long way

Two bell peppers, quartered

One summer squash halved and then quartered the long way

Rice

1 ½ cup Jasmine Rice

Three cups of water

Directions:

- To make the seasoning, mix all the seasoning ingredients together and blend evenly. Store the seasoning in an airtight jar for as much as six months.

- Rub the olive oil into each salmon filet, on both sides. Sprinkle the fillets with some of the seasonings, depending on your own flavor pallet.

- Skewer the vegetable chunks onto wooden or metal kabob skewers.

- Heat the goals on your grill, or set a gas grill to medium heat. Set the salmon directly on the grill grate. Close the grill id and cook the fish for about five mins on each side. Turn the vegetable skewers every few minutes for even heating.

- When the salmon is flaky, it is ready to come off the grill. When the veggies are tender and are starting to get brown spots, they are ready to come off the grill.

- On the stove, heat the three cups of water in a medium saucepan until boiling. Add the jasmine rice, sprinkle in a little salt, and stir the rice.

- Lower the heat on the stove down to a low simmer and cover the rice. Allow the water to simmer off and the rice to cook about fifteen to twenty minutes.

- When the rice is finished, divide onto four plates. Top the rice with salmon and serve with grilled veggies on the side.

Lentil Soup

Prep Time: Thirty mins

Cook Time: Forty-five mins

Yields: Six to Eight servings

Ingredients:

One lb. lentils, rinsed
One C onion, chopped
½ C celery, chopped
½ C carrots, chopped
One C tomatoes, peeled and diced
Two qts. Vegetable Broth
Two tbsp. olive oil
Two tsp. salt
½ tsp. coriander, ground
½ tsp. grains of paradise, ground
½ tsp. toasted cumin, ground

Directions:

- In a Dutch oven, warm the olive oil over medium heat on a stovetop. Sauté the onion, carrots, and celery together for about six to seven mins until the onions become translucent.

- Add the remaining ingredients into the Dutch oven and stir until evenly combined. Bring the heat up to high temperature and let the mixture just reach a boil.

- Return the heat to low and cover the pot with a lid. Allow simmering on low until the lentils become tender. This should take about thirty-five to forty min.

- With an emersion blender or a traditional blender, puree the soup to a creamy consistency, or your preferred consistency. Serve warm and save leftovers for up to five days in the refrigerator.

Parmesan Crusted Pork Chops (Keto)

Prep Time: Six mins

Cook Time: Twelve mins

Yields: Four servings

Ingredients:

1 ¼ lb. pork chops, boneless, fat trimmed off
Two tablespoons avocado oil

Pepper and Salt to taste

½ C parmesan cheese, grated

½ C pork rinds, crushed

½ teaspoon garlic, minced

One egg, beaten

Two teaspoons water

One tablespoon fresh parsley, chopped

½ teaspoon lemon zest

Directions:

- Allow the pork to sit out for about twenty to thirty mins, so it reaches room temperature. Season with pepper and salt. Beat the egg and water together in a bowl that is large enough for a pork chop to fit in.

- Mix the pork rinds and the parmesan together on a plate. Add the minced garlic, chopped parsley and mix in with the cheese and rinds. Mix in the lemon zest as well and stir lightly until everything is combined.

- On the stove, heat a frying pan over medium heat. Place one pork chop into the beaten egg flip it over to make sure both sides are coated. Lift from the bowl and allow the excess egg to run off. Next, put the chop onto the plate with the parmesan crust. Push it down into the topping and then flip, repeating the action on the other side to ensure the chop gets coated.

- Warm oil in the frying pan. Put the crusted chop into the pan. Bread the rest of the chops one at a time and put them in the pan. When they are all in the pan, let cook for three mins. Flip the first chop, wait a min, flip the second chop, wait a min, flip the third chop, wait one min, and then flip the last chop.

- Cook for another three minutes.

- Check the chops firmness to see if they are done. If they feel squishy when pressed, they need to be cooked longer. The pork chop is done when it feels firm.

- When done, remove the first pork chop and set it on a plate loosely covered with foil. Remove the remaining pork chops one at a time, in the order they were flipped, on min apart. Set them all on the plate and cover with foil.

- Allow the pork to sit for ten mins before serving. Serve with favorite veggie sides!

Chicken Stir Fry (Keto)

Prep Time: Ten min

Cook Time: Twelve min

Yields: Four servings

Ingredients:

Stir Fry Sauce

Four tablespoons coconut aminos
One tablespoon apple cider vinegar
Two cloves garlic, minced
One in. ginger root, grated

Stir Fry

One-pound chicken breasts, trimmed of fat, cut into strips
½ C onion, diced
Two C broccoli florets
One C button mushrooms, sliced
½ bell pepper, red or orange, chopped
½ teaspoon red pepper flakes

Two teaspoon sesame oil

Directions:

- Mix the coconut aminos, vinegar, ginger, and garlic in a bowl. Stir together and then add the chicken breast strips. Make sure the chicken is coated and let marinate for at least thirty mins.

- In a wok or sauté pan, heat the oil and then sauté the onions for 2 mins before adding the broccoli florets and peppers. Cook until the vegetables are crisp and tender.

- Remove the veggies from the pan and transfer to a bowl. Cover them with tin foil to keep warm.

- Move the chicken from the marinade to the wok or sauté pan. Add a little more oil and turn the heat up to high. Cook the chicken for three to four mins per side.

- Now add the cooked veggies back into the pan and add the remaining marinade, the mushrooms, red pepper flakes, and the sesame oil. Stir together and cook for about 3 to 4 more min.

- Once the mushrooms are cooked, remove from the stove and serve hot on a bed of white quinoa.

Snacks

Blackberry and Chia Seed Pudding

Prep Time: Five min
Cook Time: Eight hours

Yields: One serving

Ingredients:

¾ C almond milk, vanilla flavored, unsweetened
Four tbsp. chia seeds
Three tsp. filtered honey
One tsp. vanilla extract
One C fresh blackberries

Directions:

- Mash up half a cup of the blackberries with a fork in a bowl. Combine all the ingredients together in a Mason jar, including the mashed berries but excluding the remaining half cup of whole berries.

- Tighten the lid of the Mason jar and then shake the jar to get the ingredients well mixed and blended together.

- Let the Mason jar sit in the refrigerator with the pudding mix overnight.

- Scoop your pudding out of the jar and into a bowl to serve. Garnish with the whole blackberries that were set aside and drizzle with some extra honey or nuts as desired.

- Leftovers will keep when refrigerated for up to five days.

Carrot Sticks, Apple Slices, and Peanut Butter

Prep Time: Five to Ten mins.

Yields: Two to Four servings

Ingredients:

One large apple
Four medium carrots
Peanut Butter

Directions:
- Cut the apple in half and then slice each half into quarters, or sixths for thinner slices. Remove the seeds from the apple slices.

- Cut the carrots in half and then cut the halves into thirds or quarters, depending on desired slice thickness.

- Dip the apple slices and carrot sticks into peanut butter liberally and enjoy! A great snack for around the house or at work.

Fruit and Cheese Plate

Prep Time: Five Minutes

Yields: Two to Four servings

Ingredients:

Red Grapes
Green Grapes
One Pear
Cherries
Cheddar Cheese

Gouda Cheese

Brie Cheese

Quinoa Crackers

Directions:

Cut the pear in half and then slice the halves into four to six thinner slices. Remove the seeds.

Cut the cheddar, gouda, and brie cheese into square slices. Make them as thick or thin as you'd like.

Arrange the fruits and cheeses on a plate with the quinoa crackers. Enjoy with family and friends. Or pack up in a travel container and bring to work as a snack between meals.

Trail Mix (Keto)

Prep Time: Two mins

Ingredients:

One C almonds, roasted

½ C cashews

½ C sunflower seeds

¼ C coconut, shredded

Handful dried cranberries

Directions:

- Combine all ingredients in a jar or container with a lid.

- Shake the container to mix the ingredients together.

- Store in an airtight, glass container.

- A single portion is about one handful of the mix.

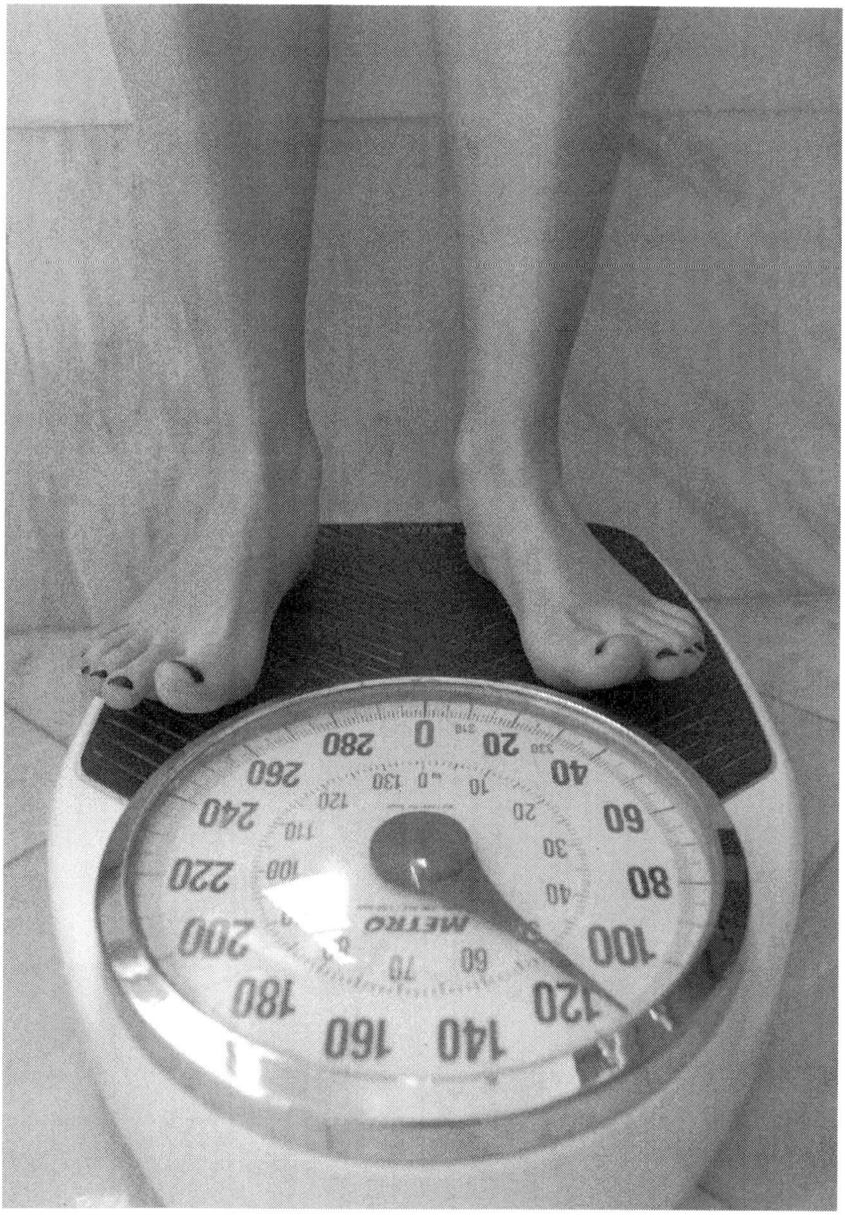
METRO

Chapter Five: Supercharge your Weight Loss

How do you supercharge your weight loss? Of course, there are a lot of ways to help stimulate your body in losing weight. Some are more intense than others, but what if there was a way to supercharge weight loss while still following the 16/8 intermittent fasting method?

Of course, there is! In this chapter, there will be details on how different approaches can help increase the weight loss potential. The keto diet is the foremost focus for supercharging weight loss in accordance with intermittent fasting!

Intermittent fasting 16/8 is an eating method that is designed to help followers lose weight by forcing the body to use up its fat stores during fasting periods. However, it can be easy to accidentally rebuild those fats stores during your eating window if you don't take care of what you eat.

Counting and restricting calories are one way to try and maximize weight loss. The only problem with that is, often times, restricting calories can lead to more hunger pains. When already operating on a 16/8 intermittent fasting plan, you want to make sure your body doesn't feel hungry all the time, or it will be harder to keep to your intermittent fasting cycle.

What really builds up the excess fat stores in the body? In previous chapters, we talked about carbohydrates being broken down during digestion, becoming glucose and powering cells. Any glucose that isn't used then becomes fat stores.

Additionally, more calories are burned when changing fat and protein into energy than it does to change carbohydrates into energy. Fewer carbohydrates make the body turn to fat and protein for energy, and the high fat and high protein diet is more satisfying. When your body is satisfied with food consumption, then you eat less in general.

So wouldn't it make more sense to limit the intake of carbohydrates rather than calories?

That is the science behind the Ketogenic Diet. Some ketogenic diet plans say to consume as little as 20 carbohydrates a day! The whole idea is to consume fewer carbohydrates and more proteins and fats. That almost sounds counterintuitive to the idea of losing weight, but it works!

What happens when fewer carbohydrates are consumed, and instead you increase the daily fat and protein intake?

Well, when the intake of carbs is reduced, the body's metabolic state changes and enters a state known as ketosis. In the ketosis metabolic state, the body becomes highly efficient in burning fat stores. Similar to how the fasting period forces the body to burn fat stores.

Additionally, ketones supply the brain with energy. When the metabolic state is in ketosis, some fat turns into those ketones in the liver. So not only do fat stores get burned faster, but some of that fat gets rerouted to supply the brain with additional energy!

While the brain has access to higher levels of ketones, you can experience better mental clarity, more brain energy or higher levels of brain function, and help keep the brain healthier. The brain is so important to the body, keeping it healthy and well 'fed' is one of the best things you can do for long term health and wellness.

That is another duel benefit that helps the body, mind, and works well with an intermittent fasting lifestyle.

There has been plenty of research to show that the keto diet has fewer risks than some stricter calorie restricting or low-fat diets, but also shows better results when it comes to actually lose weight!

The keto diet makes it possible to lose weight at a fast pace, but not starve the body. You can feel full and energized and still lose weight!

There are studies that show people following the ketogenic diet have lost 3 times more weight than people following traditional low fat or UK Diabetic recommended diets.

There is additional scientific data to suggest that following the ketogenic diet lowers the risk for heart disease, slows the growth of cancer cells, reduce symptoms of and slow down progression of Alzheimer's disease, reduce seizures for epileptic patients, improves symptoms of Parkinson's disease, improve acne conditions, reduce concussion, and also improve polycystic ovary syndrome symptoms.

Great benefits, right? And many of them are similar to, or right in line with the benefits gained from intermittent fasting!

We know that the ketogenic diet is a low carb diet. But as far as food and eating, what does that mean? What foods should be avoided? What foods can be eaten?

That's easy!

Foods to avoid on a Ketogenic Diet:

- **Sugary Foods:** cake, ice cream, smoothies, soda, candy, fruit juice, sweets, brown and white sugar, etc.

- **Beans and Legumes:** Peas, lentils, lima beans, chickpeas, kidney beans, wax beans, etc.

- **Fruit:** All fruit with the exception of small portions of berries (strawberries, blueberries, raspberries), etc.

- **Alcohol:** Most alcoholic beverages have a high carb content because of sugars, fermented fruits, and fermented grains.

- **Grains and Starches:** Wheat-based products (bread, pasta, crackers, pretzels, cereals, etc.), rice, barley, grains, etc.

- **Root Vegetables and Tubers:** Carrots, turnips, parsnips, beets, radishes, potatoes, sweet potatoes, etc.

- **Low Fat or other Diet Products:** Most low fat and diet products still contain sugars and other unhealthy fats.

- **Sugar-Free Foods:** Sugar-free means 'no sugar added' and most sugar-free foods still contain high levels of sugar alcohols. They can also be pretty highly processed.

- **Condiments and Sauces:** Many condiments have sugars and unhealthy fats. However, there are low carb condiments available.

It does seem like a slightly scary list of foods to avoid. However, when examined more carefully, most of those foods are known to be unhealthy in one way or another. At least, it is recommended that they are consumed in moderation.

Since the foods listed above are high in sugars or carbohydrates, they can produce excess amounts of glucose in the cells during digestion and cell function. The metabolic state of the body isn't allowed to enter into the target ketosis state where fat is burned more rapidly.

It can take three to four days for the body to switch into the ketosis metabolic state. That being said, going too high on the carbohydrate intake can take you out of the ketosis metabolic state much faster!

Since it is harder to enter that specific metabolic state and easier to take yourself out of it, keeping yourself in a ketosis metabolic state is the best way to optimize the keto diet benefits.

Taking a look at evolution again, before agriculture and the development of growing wheat, making bread, cultivating crops for foods, the human diet was more similar to the ketogenic diet. They didn't have access to processed wheat products, most agricultural produce, dairy, alcohol, or condiments.

While we might gain great pleasure from eating products like the aforementioned list of more modern commodities, our digestive systems didn't exactly evolve to be able to digest them. Then it makes perfect sense to try and stick to foods that are more similar to the foods early man consumed, right?

Hunter-gatherers ate meat, fish, nuts, berries, seeds, above ground vegetables that were easily available for picking. Humans were much leaner, possibly because they were nomadic and moved around a lot, as well as hunted and gathered on foot, but it also stands to reason that their diets played a role in the body fat to muscle ratio.

With an intermittent fasting plan like the 16/8 method, the body is given time to burn through those excess fat stores. To supercharge the weight loss and fat burning, eating a diet that prevents additional buildup of fat stores, like the keto diet, means that fat will keep burning but not keep accumulating.

That sounds like a win/win situation for optimizing both the keto diet and intermittent fasting! If weight loss is your primary goal with intermittent fasting, following a keto diet incongruence will only help!

With such a long list of foods that can't be eaten on the keto diet, what about foods that can be eaten?

Foods that can be eaten on the keto diet:

- **Meat:** Steak, red meat, sausage, bacon, ham, chicken, turkey, duck

- **Cheese:** Cheddar, cream, mozzarella, blue cheese, goat cheese, other unprocessed cheeses

- **Nuts and Seeds:** Walnuts, flax seeds, pumpkin seeds, almonds, chia seeds, etc.

- **Fatty Fish:** Trout, salmon, tuna, mackerel, white fish

- **Condiments:** Salt, black pepper, healthy herbs and spices
- **Low-carb Vegetables:** Tomatoes, green vegetables, peppers, onions, etc.

- **Healthy Oils:** Olive oil, avocado oil, coconut oil

- **Avocados:** Fresh avocados or avocados in guacamole

When comparing the list of foods that can be eaten on the keto diet, a lot of them are also listed in previous chapters with the whole foods recommended to have in stock when following your 16/8 intermittent fasting method.

In terms of matching what primitive man ate, the Paleo diet is definitely closer to the original 'caveman' diet of the hunter-gatherer. The keto diet provides a similar evolutionary diet as well as some more modern variety and modern benefits. Modern society and lifestyles aren't the same as back in the hunter-gatherer days, so following the same kind of diet might not be ideal. Due to our jobs, families, forms of transportation, and so forth, humans on a large scale aren't as active as they once were.

That being said, a diet like a keto diet is a modern diet for the humans of today!

For the keto diet, having meals and snacks that are limited to only a few ingredients is ideal. You'll notice that a lot of the recipes for intermittent fasting meal ideas follow similar logic of limited ingredients and whole foods.

Limited ingredients refer to the idea that a meal can be as few as one to three ingredients. While sticking to limited ingredient meals and snacks isn't a requirement for 16/8 intermittent fasting or the keto diet, it is another way to increase your nutritional benefit but decrease your carbohydrate intake.

Think about it, the more ingredients a single meal has, the higher it will be in carbohydrates and calories, especially if it includes foods that are on the 'non-keto approved' list.

For keto diet enthusiasts, there are some meal ideas listed below that could be used during your non-fasting eating window, depending on if you have an early, midday, or late eating window.

Breakfast

One: bacon, tomatoes, and eggs

Two: omelet with egg, basil, goat cheese, and tomato

Three: Milkshake that follows ketogenic guidelines

Four: Plain, sugar-free yogurt mixed with cocoa powder, peanut butter, and stevia (low carb sweetener)

Five: Egg omelet with ham, cheese, and veggies

Six: Egg omelet with salsa, peppers, salt and pepper, onion, and avocado

Seven: Fried eggs with mushrooms and bacon

Lunch

One: Burger topped with cheese, salsa, and guacamole

Two: Slices of ham and cheese with mixed nuts

Three: Stir-fried beef and veggies in coconut oil

Four: Mixed nuts and celery sticks with salsa and guacamole for dipping

Five: Shrimp salad topped with avocado and seasoned with olive oil

Six: Milkshake with almond milk, cocoa powder, peanut butter, and stevia

Seven: Chicken salad with feta crumbles and olive oil for dressing

Dinner

One: Salmon and asparagus cooked in butter

Two: Roasted vegetables, meatballs with cheddar cheese

Three: Stuffed chicken with cream cheese and pesto, side of vegetables

Four: Bun free burger topped with an egg, bacon, and cheese

Five: Whitefish fillet with a fried egg and spinach cooked in coconut oil

Six: Pork chops sprinkled with parmesan cheese, steamed broccoli, and a side salad

Seven: Steak with fried eggs and a small side salad

The keto recommended meals are high in protein and have enough calories to keep the body full and energized, but limited carbohydrates to prevent glucose build up. These kinds of meals are ideal for getting you into your ketosis metabolic state. Not to mention, they are easy to prepare and make. Limited ingredient meals and snacks cut back on food costs and meal prep time. Use more of that time and money for something else you love!

Since the 16/8 intermittent fasting plan is designed around one large meal or two small meals and snacks, it only makes sense to include some Keto snacks along with meal ideas. This will ensure you have everything you need to get started on a supercharged intermittent fasting lifestyle!

Keto Snacks

Cheese Slices

Mixed nuts and seeds

Cheese slices with olives

Dark chocolate, 90% or higher

Plain, full fat, yogurt mixed with cocoa powder and peanut butter (or other preferred nut butter)

One to Two hard boiled or soft boiled eggs

Almond milk milkshake with cocoa powder and peanut butter (or preferred nut butter)

Celery with guacamole and salsa

Strawberries with cream

Ripe avocado

Snacks that are comprised of a few small ingredients, and are in small portions, like just a handful of nuts, are ideal for both keto and intermittent fasting plans. Snacks that include cheeses, yogurt, milk, and nuts and seeds are especially recommended as they are higher in protein and fat, and rich in nutrients. This will help you keep feeling full and providing your body with the nutrients to prevent unhealthy eating habits from developing.

Weight loss is a struggle for a lot of people. How can it not be with how easily available unhealthy foods are? One of the reasons that it is recommended to eat whole, clean foods, instead of processed foods while on an intermittent fasting plan is because so many processed foods are full of preservatives.

What is a preservative then? Well, a preservative is an ingredient added to processed foods to make them last longer or have a longer shelf life.

Take fast food hamburgers, for instance. Most of us are familiar with the old studies that were done on fast food burgers that showed how, after months, or even years, the burgers were still untouched by mold.

This phenomenon occurs when processed foods are covered in preservatives. These chemicals are literally designed to keep mold and bacteria away so foods can last longer.

There are several theories about how that changes the way our bodies can digest food. If a food item is so covered in preservatives that mold doesn't recognize it as food, how can our bodies recognize it as food? If the digestive system doesn't process an item like food, then it isn't extracting the proper nutrients.

Additionally, if a burger doesn't 'break down' or get decomposed by mold, then it stands to reason that the digestive system will also have trouble breaking this food down. If it can't be digested properly, then nutrients don't get received by the body. More than that, what is extracted from the preservative covered food doesn't always get translated as proper nutrients, and it can become excess fat.

Keeping in mind that highly processed foods, such as bread, cakes, fast foods, instant box meals, cheese sauces, etc. are covered in preservatives, sticking to whole, clean foods is the best way to go for weight loss purposes.

These foods provide the body with nutrients and less waste that might cause difficulties in digestion, leading to additional fat build up.

So, whether you simply follow the 16/8 intermittent fasting method, or follow the keto diet as well, including as many unprocessed foods into your eating window schedule is another path to maximizing your weight loss potential!

Another way to help supercharge your weight loss plan is exercise. With the combined benefits of both the 16/8 intermittent fasting plan and the keto diet, fat stores are going to be getting burned quicker by default. However, adding in some physical labor and getting your body's cells to work more will also require them to use more energy.

Once they use up available glucose, if they are still being prompted to work through physical activity, then they will turn to fat stores.

Now, physical activity doesn't have to mean a rigorous workout routine. If your body is already working to burn fat stores because you are consuming fewer carbohydrates and you are following the 16/8 intermittent fasting cycle, then it won't take much to burn additional fat stores.

Going for a ten to fifteen-minute walk in the morning or evening can boost your weight loss potential. So, can doing a twenty-minute yoga routine or a gentle weight lifting routine.

Please note that if you are going to push your body rigorously with working out and physical activity, it might make you feel hungrier as you will be burning through calories faster.

Here again, we see how the keto diet and the 16/8 intermittent fasting method complement each other. Calories aren't limited in the keto diet, so exercise shouldn't interfere with the fasting cycle as much as if you were limiting calories and keeping up physical exercise.

Still, that exercise will prompt the cells to burn through more glucose and fat stores. Sticking to low carbohydrate meals will yield the greatest weight loss benefit.

If you are new to fasting, it is recommended that you allow your body to adjust to the fasting cycle before incorporating more intense workouts and physical activity. Make sure to drink plenty of water, especially when working out or exercising lightly. This will help reduce the risk of negative side effects.

When taking on a new exercise routine, it is also recommended that you ease into the exercise, just like easing into intermittent fasting. Give your body the time to adjust and acclimate before overdoing it. If you do too much too quickly, you run the risk of causing damage.

The whole idea behind intermittent fasting, the keto diet, and regular exercise is to benefit the body, lose weight, increase overall health, and develop healthy eating habits. Not cause damage! Be conscious of how you are treating your body.

Going back to the keto diet, there are a few different types of keto diets that can be followed. Different types follow slightly different food restrictions, but overall, they are based on limiting and lowering carbohydrate intake.

Types of keto diets:

- Standard Keto Diet (SKD)
- Cyclical Ketogenic Diet (CKD)
- Targeted Ketogenic Diet (TKD)
- High-Protein Ketogenic Diet

The SKD plan functions on a very low carb basis with moderate protein and a high-fat content diet. The percentage breakdown is about 75 percent fat, 5 percent carbs, and 20 percent protein.

The CKD plan follows the same similar idea as a 5:2 intermittent fasting plan, although it doesn't innately include fasting. The idea is to spend 5 days in a ketogenic state and then follow those 5 days with 2 days of a high carb diet.

The TKD plan encourages you to intermittently add carbohydrates around your exercise and workout routine.

The High-protein ketogenic diet plan is in many ways similar to the SKD; however, it incorporates a higher percentage of protein. The breakdown is more along the lines of 5 percent carbohydrates, 60 percent fat, and 35 percent protein.

In the case of including a keto diet in with a 16/8 intermittent fasting plan, the Standard and High Protein keto diet are probably the easiest to incorporate. If trying to balance intermittent fasting with intermittent low carb days, it might get confusing.

Some other benefits of the keto diet are in regards to the treatment of diabetes and prediabetes. The fact that the ketogenic diet promotes rapid weight loss helps reduce the impact of developing type 2 diabetes as weight is a significant factor. In one study, participants following the keto diet lost 24.4 pounds while the higher carbohydrate group only lost 15.2 pounds.

Considering that the weight loss was much more significant in the keto diet group, it can be a great preventative for type 2 diabetes. One study even found that the keto diet improved people who followed its insulin sensitivity by a huge 75 percent!

Studies with individuals who have type 2 diabetes that is also following the ketogenic diet found that a third of the participants were able to completely stop diabetic medication use!

There is also evidence to suggest that the ketogenic diet can help endurance athletes, such as cyclists and runners. The ketogenic diet seems to offer them benefits during their training. When used over time, the keto diet helps the muscle to fat ratio in the body. The amount of oxygen that your body can use while it's working out, although it isn't the best diet for peak performance.

Some of the side effects that come with the keto diet are low blood sugar, indigestion, or constipation. Rarely the keto diet can lead to increased acid levels in the body or kidney stones. A few other side effects sometimes include headache, weakness, bad breath, fatigue, and irritability. These are symptoms of the keto flu.

If you already have heart disease, epilepsy, diabetes, or a preexisting condition, it might be best to have a doctor guide you through starting the keto diet and ensure that you do it right.

As with the 16/8 intermittent fasting method, ease into the keto diet, and allow your body to adjust properly to the changes you are making. If you have any questions or concerns or feel any of these side effects, please contact your doctor or healthcare professional.

Alright, so now we have covered the individual benefits of both the keto diet and the 16/8 intermittent fasting method. We've also gone over the foods that are ideal for both methods and some of the science behind how they work. This chapter did discuss how the keto diet can jump start your 16/8 intermittent fasting cycle for increased weight loss potential.

What about mutual benefits? Does intermittent fasting complement the keto diet as well?

Actually, yes, it does!

Is that so surprising? The more research that comes out about weight loss and the best methods for achieving weight loss goals rapidly, the more eating plans and diets are emerging that do actually work off of each other to provide greater benefit.

Intermittent fasting can actually put the body into a ketosis metabolic state faster than the three to four days it takes while just following the keto diet! Getting to a ketosis metabolic state faster will encourage weight loss benefits to kick in sooner. Who doesn't want that?

While research on combining the two methods is limited, based on the science behind both, as well as the goals and health benefits of both, it is clear to see how they can work together. The synergistic benefits are there in science. Even if the research doesn't combine the two methods, since they do share so many studied and reviewed benefits, their congruence is almost obvious!

The keto diet benefits again show similar impacts as the benefits of intermittent fasting. These two methods of weight loss complement each other greatly. Granted, the keto diet is designed to be a short term weight loss method and not a long term health solution.

However, the 16/8 intermittent fasting method can be used in the long term for subtler weight loss or as a healthy lifestyle change. Using the keto diet with an intermittent fasting plan is a great way to drop weight fast. Once the weight is off, introducing a higher percentage of carbohydrates can continue to promote health benefits without becoming potentially harmful to the body.

As with any change in lifestyle or eating habits, there is a potential risk, especially if you have a preexisting condition. If you have a history of eating disorders, it is not recommended that you try the keto diet. Just like with intermittent fasting, limiting the consumption of carbohydrates can unintentionally encourage unhealthy eating habits. Your goal is to maintain health in a way that the body doesn't suffer!

There you have it. Go ahead and get your 16/8 intermittent fasting plan kick-started with the added benefits of combining with the keto diet! Get rapid results that you can see and feel! Maximize your health and wellness and start to bring through your fat stores! Drop pounds and waist circumference for an overall healthier lifestyle!

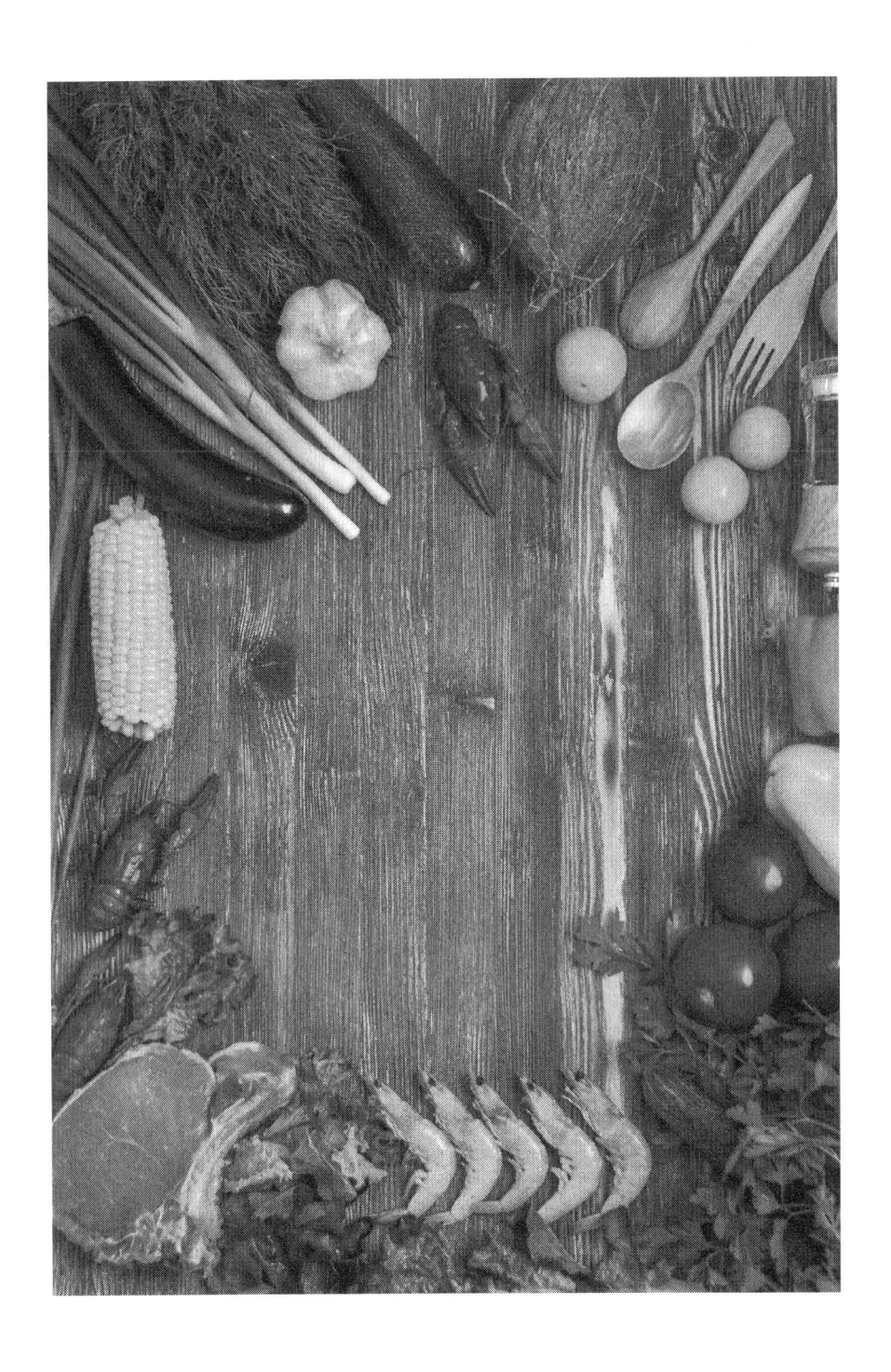

Chapter Six: Extras

You made it! You have successfully navigated through the nitty-gritty information of following a successful 16/8 intermittent fasting plan and how to supercharge it with the keto diet! Wow! You must be really excited to start pursuing your new weight loss plan. You should be!

Before we wrap up, there are some additional tips, tricks, and hacks that can help ensure success with your 16/8 intermittent fasting plan with or without the keto diet add on.

Some of these tips have been touched on before, but now they will be elaborated on in greater detail. This chapter should be a great reference to have while you are getting yourself set up and started on weight loss!

Hydration

What is hydration, and why is it so important?

Well, hydration refers to the water content and levels in your body. The human body is comprised of about 80 percent water. That sounds crazy, right? Well, it isn't. Every cell, tissue, organ, and intricate part of the body has water content and relies on water to keep itself functioning properly. It is used to help with waste elimination, maintaining body temperature and homeostasis, and even to help your joints stay lubricated.

Water gets lost from our body every day. Whether it is through perspiration, waste elimination, or other subtle water excretion processes, the human body constantly loses water. Which means we should be taking care to replenish it!

The 'general' assumption is to drink somewhere between six and eight 8 oz cups of water a day. This is fairly average water intake. However, not everyone needs the same amount of water.

A lot of water can be consumed through foods you eat. Certain raw vegetables have high water content, and when eaten, they replenish the body with water. If you get a lot of water through your diet, you may not need to drink as much.

Some people are more active or just perspire more due to genetics or body mass index. Heavy perspires may need to drink more water to keep themselves hydrated.

Dehydration can be dangerous. A light headache and nausea are not so serious side effects, but severe dehydration can lead to riskier or life-threatening situations.

Okay, so how does water relate to your 16/8 intermittent fasting regime? Well, for 16 hours a day, you won't be eating. That means you won't be consuming water through the foods you eat. You might be light or moderately active during your 16 hour fasting period, or be in high temperatures with dry or humid climates that contribute to dehydration.

Drinking water during your fasting cycle means that you aren't consuming additional calories or carbohydrates. However, you are keeping yourself hydrated when other sources of water are unavailable.

Additionally, drinking water can help keep cravings from popping up or help satiate minor hunger pangs that could cause discomfort during your fasting cycle. Especially when you first start, and your body is adjusting.

Since water doesn't have calories or carbohydrates, it is also a desirable beverage during your eating window. As strange as it sounds, it is possible to over drink water and over saturates your body with water, so definitely be aware of that. Generally speaking, water during your fasting period or eating window is an acceptable choice of beverage.

During your eating window, you can even look into using low carb drink mix packets that can be added to water for additional flavor. As a somewhat tasteless substance, it can be nice to spice up a glass of water with a flavor packet!

Coffee

A lot of people drink coffee. Coffee itself has become a sort of lifestyle commodity. Coffee comes in so many forms, styles, and even flavors. Most people do have a daily routine that includes coffee of some kind.

When considering coffee and your 16/8 intermittent fasting method, during your eating window, coffee with milk and sweeteners is fair game! Remember that any additives have calories and carbohydrates, so moderation is key.

What about during the fasting cycle? Well, coffee can still be consumed, but without any additives. Some people can't handle the harshness of black coffee and may not want to try this.

There are many different coffee roasts available on the market now. Some are even flavored! When looking into the health benefits of coffee that will complement the 16/8 intermittent fasting plan, let's take a closer look at Dark Roast Coffee.

What is dark roast coffee?

Dark roast coffee is often described as coffee with a full, intense flavor that can be bittersweet, bold, and even smoky. Essentially, dark roast coffee beans are roasted to an internal temperature that is about 50-100 degrees F higher than light roast beans. The higher temperatures change the composition of the sugars, caffeine, and flavor of the beans.

Often times, dark roast coffee can be easier going down black than light roast, which means it is an excellent no calorie beverage during fasting periods.

A dark roast tends to have a little less caffeine than a light roast, but anything with caffeine should be drunk before or during your eating window.

Dark roast coffees have also shown greater health benefits than light roast coffee. First off, some people with sensitive gastrointestinal tracts that can't drink coffee easily have found that they can drink black dark roast coffee with little to no irritation.

Research has been done into Molecular Food and Nutrition that has indicated dark roast coffee can restore Vitamin E, red blood cells, and glutathione much more effectively than the average light roast coffee. Further research in that study showed that dark roast coffee showed a decrease in body weight in pre-obese individuals.

Wow! Who knew that dark roast coffee could assist in weight loss? That sounds even better when we are talking about beverages that can be drunk during a fasting period on an intermittent fasting plan designed for weight loss!

While any black coffee is acceptable to drink during your fasting cycle, the dark roast has some better health benefits that actually align with a weight loss goal!

Tea

Some people just aren't coffee drinkers. There is nothing wrong with that! There are other options, such as tea. Tea is another readily available beverage that is very low calorie when consumed with no additives.

Just like coffee, tea can come in so many forms and styles with different flavors, serving methods, and dressings.

Tea with no additives is an approved fasting period beverage because it is low calorie, and most tears are also low carb unless they are fruit-based flavors.

There is one tea type that is right in line with some superfoods and has extraordinary benefits on the body and mind. It used to be a secret but has slowly been gaining more attention. This particular tea is absolutely perfect to work alongside your 16/8 intermittent fasting method!
Green Tea. Most everyone has heard of green tea in one form or another, such as macha, or a green tea Frappuccino, or as a flavor in ice cream even!

We are talking about just plain old loose leaf or in a bag green tea! It is quite literally one of the healthiest beverages on the planet. Whether you drink it warm in a mug or have it iced, the benefits of green tea are huge! And, not surprisingly, go hand in hand with many of the benefits and goals of the 16/8 intermittent fasting method!

Some of the health benefits of green tea include:

- Improved brain function
- Increase fat burning
- Improved physical performance
- Reduce the risk of some cancers
- Lowers risk of Alzheimer's and Parkinson's
- Kills bacteria
- Improves dental health
- Decreases risk of infection
- Reduces the risk of type 2 Diabetes
- Lowers cardiovascular disease risk
- Help weight loss
- Prevent obesity
- Increase longevity

Wow! A lot of those benefits have already been discussed in terms of 16/8 intermittent fasting as well as the keto diet! Imagine all that packed into just one cup of tea. Incredible, right?

So what is it about green tea that makes it so healthy?

First of all, green tea is packed full of nutrients in the form of bioactive compounds. One of the most prominent compounds in green tea is ECGC, or Epigallocatechin Gallate, which has been studied extensively as a treatment for various diseases.

Green tea also contains antioxidants and minerals beneficial to good health.

Green tea contains caffeine. Lower levels than coffee, but still enough to stimulate the brain. Between the caffeine and amino acid in green tea called L-theanine green tea actually assists in brain function. It increases dopamine, has an anti-anxiety effect, and increasing the alpha waves in the brain.

The caffeine and L-theanine work together synergistically to overall improve brain function.

These brain benefits aren't just for short term; they can extend to long term brain protection from neurodegenerative diseases.

Most weight loss supplements include green tea. That is because green tea has been proven in human trials to increase the metabolic rate and induce fat burning at a faster rate.

With an increased metabolic rate, fat is burned quicker. Not to mention, green tea-induced weight loss has also been known to target the abdominal fat stores, reducing belly fat and waist circumference.

The antioxidants in green tea have been known to reduce the risks of breast cancer, prostate cancer, and colorectal cancer. Green tea drinkers are 20 to 30 percent less likely to develop breast cancer, 48 percent less likely to develop prostate cancer, and 42 percent less likely to develop colorectal cancer. Those are pretty big odds!

The catechins that are contained in green tea have multiple biological effects within the body. Influenza is a nasty virus and somewhat common. Green tea catechins can actually inhibit the development of influenza viruses, and others, which also reduces the risk of infection.

Then there is something as common as mutant strains of Streptococcus which contribute to oral bacteria, plaque, tooth decay, and gum infection. Guess what can fight and reduce the growth of mutant Streptococcus? Yup! Green tea! That means green tea can even combat bad breath.

Green tea has the effect of lowering blood sugar levels in the body. Green tea drinkers are 18 percent to 42 percent less likely to develop type 2 diabetes. Whether or not green tea can help reduce the use of diabetic medication was not part of that particular study. It may be more functional as a preventative.

Cardiovascular disease is often caused when LDL cholesterol and triglycerides are oxidized. Green tea helps reduce oxidation levels. Green tea drinkers are known to have 31 percent less of a chance to develop potentially life-threatening cardiovascular disease. Since cardiovascular disease is one of the most common killers today, that is a huge benefit!

Since green tea can reduce cardiovascular disease and cancer risks, it has been known to increase longevity for the body. As a whole, green tea has also been known to decrease the mortality rate for any cause by 23 percent in women and 12 percent in men.

This is absolutely amazing information. To have a beverage that can be consumed during fasting periods and your designated eating window that provides similar and different benefits to your 16/8 intermittent fasting plan is incredible.
Of course, green tea isn't a cure-all, but it certainly does give other low calorie and low carbohydrate drinks a run for their money in the health department!

How do you make the perfect cup of green tea? Many people shy away from green tea because it can have a bitter taste or a strong aftertaste. Fortunately, there is a way to brew the perfect cup of green tea.

First, you want to make sure you have the right amount of tea. A standard tea bag is fine for an average sized mug. If you are using loose leaf tea, about one teaspoon of the tea leaves per six ounces of water is a good ratio.

The water should be fresh and cool, tap, spring, or filtered. Distilled water isn't ideal for tea as it can provide a flat flavor.

For green tea, you want to bring the water just short of boiling, roughly 160 degrees to 180 degrees F.

In a mug, you should have your tea bag or loose-leaf tea in an infuser. Pour the hot water over the tea and cover with a plate. Allow the tea too steep for one to three minutes. Depending on how strong you like your tea, you might want to taste it in thirty-second intervals to avoid brewing.

Once brewed to the desired flavor, uncover and take the teabag or infuser out. There is your perfect cup of green tea. During your eating window, sweeten with a little milk and/or honey if you like.

Of course, there are hundreds of varieties of tea. Black tea, white tea, herbal tea, oolong tea, green tea, twig tea, and then each of those is broken down into several other categories of tea like Earl Grey, Irish Breakfast, Darjeeling, and different flavors too.

Tea is a great low-calorie beverage in any form or flavor. If you are looking to maximize your health and weight loss benefits with a beverage that keeps on giving during your fasting period, green tea is a great option!

Decaf vs. Caffeine

Most coffees and teas come with decaf and caffeinated options. Generally, people like to drink their caffeine in the morning or afternoon to help wake them up or give them a second wind to get through the day.

When this section is referring to caffeinated or non-caffeinated beverages, it is specifically referring to tea and coffee.

With a 16/8 intermittent fasting plan, it is recommended that you drink any caffeinated beverages in the morning or at the beginning of your eating window. Decaf beverages should be consumed when you're eating window closes.

There are a few reasons for this. First off, if you have your fasting schedule set up so that you will sleep through a portion of your fasting cycle, then caffeine has the potential to keep you awake longer. If the goal is to sleep through most of your fasting cycle, try not to tempt fate by drinking beverages that could keep you up.

Additionally, caffeine stimulates the mind and body. If you are in a stimulated zone, your body will be more sensitive, and you can start feeling more intensely hungry.

If you don't like decaf beverages, sticking to water once you're eating window closes is a good plan. If you don't like caffeinated beverages, then you don't really need to worry.

There are some different benefits for decaf and caffeinated beverages, though.

Let's look at what caffeine has to offer in terms of benefits first. Well, it can stimulate the metabolic process to encourage fat burning. However, this is usually a temporary effect, and once your body is used to caffeine, it stops responding to the metabolic stimulation and the benefit goes away.

Some other benefits of caffeinated beverages include:

- Improved mood
- Better reaction time
- Increased memory and mental function
- Enhanced athletic performance
- Reduce depression
- Reduced risk of cirrhosis of the liver

Many of these benefits, such as mood, brain function and memory, and athletic performance, are going to be based on the body's tolerance of caffeine. If you drink caffeine every day, your body will most likely be acclimated to the presence of caffeine, and the benefits won't be as prominent or long term.

Caffeine is a stimulant that can and does reduce tiredness, increases alertness, and increases energy levels. However, caffeine is a substance that stimulates parts of the brain and body to feel less tired and more alert. It doesn't actually provide the body and mind with energy sources or better neural pathways.

Drinking caffeine can contribute to insomnia, especially if drunk closer to your designated sleep time. If consumed regularly and in large quantities, if you miss a day or stop drinking caffeine, your body will feel sluggish, and you'll have headaches. This is essentially your body 'coming down' to its natural levels of energy and alertness. Consumption of caffeine is recommended in moderation.

What about decaffeinated beverages? Well, they kind of have a bad reputation, unfortunately. Beverages such as herbal tea, which are innately decaf, are often naturally sweet, flavorful, and enjoyable.

Decaf coffee is the culprit when it comes to the negative stigma. However, it is an undeserved reputation because decaf coffee definitely has benefits. Some might even be more desirable than caffeinated coffee benefits.

While decaf coffee isn't one hundred percent caffeine free, it is drastically lower in caffeine than regular coffee. However, decaf coffee is loaded with nutrients and antioxidants that benefit overall health.

Decaf coffee benefits include:

- Decreased risk of Type 2 Diabetes
- Reduced risk of premature death
- Reduction in acid reflux and heartburn

The above examples have been studied with both regular coffee and decaf coffee. The general scientific consensus is that decaf is better at reducing acid reflux and heartburn than regular coffee. Decaffeinated coffee drinkers have also shown a higher decrease in the development of Type 2 diabetes than regular coffee drinkers.

Premature death is a pretty vague and broad term. However, decaffeinated coffee has shown decreases in unexpected premature death with its drinkers, more so than regular coffee.

Alright, so both caffeinated and decaffeinated coffees and teas have benefits. Remember that when following the 16/8 intermittent fasting method, try to drink caffeinated beverages before or during your eating window. Reserve decaffeinated beverages for after your eating window.

Exercise

When it comes to exercise, every human needs some kind of exercise. Human bodies were designed for movement. Unfortunately, so many jobs, forms of transportation, and modern activities (video games, social media, etc.) encourage people to stay in one place, sit, or lie down for extended periods of time. While rest is important, those long-term periods of stagnation are detrimental to the body!

Movement equals health. Exercise is movement. So many people think of exercise as rigorous weight lifting at the gym, or long, intense runs on a treadmill.

Fortunately, exercise is pretty diverse. For thousands of years, it has been known the movement and exercise stimulate the metabolism and encourage fat burning as well as an increase in muscle tone.

But exercise can be as simple as a twenty-minute walk in the morning, taking a five-minute stretch break at your desk at work to get your body moving, lifting weights, doing yoga, jogging, cycling, hiking, skiing, swimming, the list just keeps going and going.

Your body was meant to move, so move it!

That being said, an exercise in accordance with your 16/8 intermittent fasting method will only encourage your body to burn more fat! If you are heavily athletic, make sure to balance the appropriate amount of calories with exercise as well as hydration.

When speaking of overall health and wellness, exercise and movement can really only help. Don't push yourself, start slow, and allow your body to get used to movement and exercise. Just like when you start intermittent fasting, ease into exercise. Stick with it! You might be amazed at how good your body feels.

Exercise can also decrease cravings during your fasting period. It gives your mind and body something else to work on, as well as jumpstarts your body into burning fat stores. While those fat stores are actively burning, you won't feel as hungry. Your cells have already turned to a different source of energy.

The increase in muscle mass and decrease in body fat will also be noticeable as you exercise with your 16/8 intermittent fasting lifestyle.

Tips specific to 16/8 Intermittent Fasting

The tips listed above are great in regards to maximizing your health benefits and weight loss overall, as well as with a 16/8 intermittent fasting plan.

However, there are some life hacks that will make your 16/8 intermittent fasting experience easier and more enjoyable, as well as more successful!

These tips include:

- Eating healthy foods
- Drink lots of water
- Exercise
- Avoid artificially flavored drinks
- Keep busy during fasting periods
- Get plenty of sleep
- Control your stress
- Fasting means Zero

The first three tips on our list have already been covered in varying detail. Let's take a look at the rest of the list.

Avoiding artificially flavored beverages like sodas and energy drinks is a good idea. Most of them are very high in sugars and carbohydrates. The ones that are 'sugar-free' or 'low sugar' often include artificial sweeteners that are not healthy in the least.

During your fasting cycle, depending on when you decide to schedule it around sleep, there will probably be somewhere between 8 and 10 hours that you are awake and fasting. Keeping busy and productive helps stimulate the fat burning, but also takes your mind off food and eating.

Try taking a walk, keeping a journal, catching up on chores, read, anything that can keep your mind and body buys.

Sleep is imperative to health and body and mind function. Did you know that you burn calories and fat during sleep? Sleep also allows your body to repair itself and helps reduce stress. All important factors for healthy, especially if you are changing your lifestyle with intermittent fasting.

Stress is one of the major triggers for overeating, binging, and emotional eating. Stress can also lead to a lack of sleep. When emotional eating, we tend to focus on unhealthy foods. Try using calming essential oils, like lavender. Drink chamomile tea, or take a relaxing walk on your own.

Discipline is also important. It can be hard to discipline yourself into not eating during your fasting hours. Try an affirmation, like verbally reminding yourself that fasting means no food. Write it on post-it notes and sticks that on your fridge or cabinet. Verbal and visual reminders will help you form that disciplinary mindset.

Alright! Now you have everything you need to dive into our 16/8 intermittent fasting cycle and start maximizing your health and weight loss, including additional tips and hacks to ensure success. Good luck!

Conclusion

Thank you for reading through to the end of this book, *Intermittent Fasting 16/8*! Hopefully, you have found the information provided in this chapter helpful, and it was able to provide you with all of the tools you need to get started with your intermittent fasting and rapid weight loss plan.

The next step is to determine what you want your intermittent 16/8 fasting cycle to be. Then go out and fill your pantry with clean, whole foods that will benefit your body with intermittent fasting or by following the Ketogenic Diet alongside your intermittent fasting lifestyle!

You should have the preliminary information you need to get started with making your own snacks and meals to maximize your weight loss potential and limit your carbohydrates and fat store accumulation.

Get ready to feel the health benefits and the amazing changes in your body as you utilize a 16/8 intermittent fasting plan. Shed weight and belly fat quickly and improve your overall health as well as reduce your risk for certain diseases long term.

There are plenty of other sources of information about intermittent fasting and the ketogenic diet. Thank you for choosing this book and using it as your guide to getting started! There is always more to learn and always more information, but the chapters are written hear should offer you the basics for getting started and put to rest any concerns you may have had.

Finally, if this book proved helpful and the information useful, a review on Amazon is always appreciated!

COSTA Password.
Alfie Sam £4591 /

McDonalds Password

~~AlSamLin 8491 3/8 /~~
Al Sam 1948 /

Printed in Great Britain
by Amazon